MANAG

CHRONIC OBSTRUCTIVE PULMONARY DISEASE

SECOND EDITION

PETER J BARNES

SP
SCIENCE
PRESS

Published by Science Press Ltd, 34–42 Cleveland Street, London W1T 4LB, UK

Reprinted in 2003

http://current-science-group.com/

British Library Cataloguing in Publication Data.

A catalogue record for this book is available from the British Library.

ISBN 1-85873-932-2

Project editors: Alexandra Holliday and Clare Wheatcroft
Designer: Simon Banister
Production: Adrienne Hanratty

Printed in Italy by Offset Print Veneta S.r.l.

Contents

Author biography

Professor Peter Barnes is Professor of Thoracic Medicine and Head of Respiratory Medicine at the National Heart and Lung Institute, Imperial College, and an Honorary Consultant Physician at Royal Brompton Hospital, London, UK. He qualified at Cambridge and Oxford Universities. After working in Oxford he moved to London in 1974 and trained in respiratory and general medicine. He undertook research at the Royal Postgraduate Medical School and obtained a DM degree in 1982. He spent a year at the Cardiovascular Research Institute in San Francisco and returned to a Consultant post at Hammersmith Hospital, London. He was awarded a DSc from Oxford University in 1986. In 1995 he was appointed to the first Chair in Clinical Pharmacology at the National Heart and Lung Institute and in 1987 was appointed Head of Thoracic Medicine. He now heads Respiratory Medicine at Imperial College with over 200 research workers, making it the largest respiratory department in Europe.

Professor Barnes runs a large and active multidisciplinary group of over 50 researchers exploring the mechanisms and treatment of asthma and more recently COPD. He has linked molecular and cell biology to clinical studies in order to understand the inflammatory process in airway disease and to understand the mechanisms of action of currently used drugs. His research is particularly concerned with the role of transcription factors and signal transduction pathways in regulation of chronic airway inflammation and the molecular mechanisms of corticosteroid action. He has also pioneered the use of non-invasive markers to monitor lung inflammation, which has enabled research into inflammatory mechanisms to be extended to patients with severe disease.

Professor Barnes has published about 600 papers in peer-reviewed journals and has written, edited or co-edited over 30 books on airway diseases and lung pharmacology. He has delivered several named lectures, including the prestigious Amberson Lecture at the American Thoracic Society. He serves on the editorial boards of over 20 international journals, including the *New England Journal of Medicine, American Journal of Physiology* and *Thorax,* is an Associate Editor of the *American Journal of Respiratory and Critical Care Medicine*. He was previously the founding editor of *Pulmonary Pharmacology* and Associate Editor of the *European Respiratory Journal, British Journal of Clinical Pharmacology* and *Journal of Applied Physiology*. He is the Chairman of the National Asthma Taskforce in the UK and also serves on several national and international advisory boards.

Chapter 1

Epidemiology and mechanisms

Chronic obstructive pulmonary disease (COPD), sometimes called chronic obstructive airways disease, is a major cause of morbidity and mortality throughout the world. Despite the fact that it is increasing in prevalence, the disease has received relatively little attention from the medical profession or from the pharmaceutical industry. The importance of COPD has been recognised, and this has resulted in formulation of treatment guidelines in many countries and an investment in research. Recently, the World Health Organization (WHO) and the US National Institutes of Health formed a Global Initiative for Chronic Obstructive Lung Disease (GOLD), resulting in the formulation of international guidelines for the management of COPD that can be applied throughout the world [1].

Definitions

Definitions are important to distinguish COPD from asthma and to characterize differences in smoking-related diseases of the airways. GOLD has defined COPD as 'a disease state characterized by airflow limitation that is not fully reversible. The airflow limitation is usually progressive and associated with an abnormal inflammatory response of the lungs to noxious particles and gases'.

Several terms are in common usage:

Chronic simple bronchitis is defined by a productive cough on most days for at least three months for at least two consecutive years and cannot be attributed to other pulmonary or cardiac causes. It is a consequence of mucus hyperplasia, resulting in hypersecretion of mucus. *Chronic simple bronchitis is not necessarily related to airway obstruction.*

Chronic obstructive bronchitis is due to obstruction of peripheral airways as a result of an inflammatory response (bronchiolitis).

Emphysema is a pathological diagnosis characterized by destruction of alveolar walls, resulting in abnormal and permanent enlargement of airspaces and loss of lung elasticity, with consequent obstruction of peripheral airways.

COPD is defined physiologically as chronic airflow obstruction and may be due to a mixture of emphysema and peripheral airway obstruction from chronic bronchitis. This is reflected by a reduction in maximum expiratory flow and slow forced emptying of the lungs. Extensive pulmonary damage occurs before the patient is aware of symptoms, such as exertional dyspnoea, because of the slowly progressive nature of the airflow obstruction and various coping manoeuvres. There may be a small degree of reversibility in airway obstruction (<15%), in contrast to the more than 15% reversibility and variability in the airflow obstruction in asthma.

Chronic hypoxia occurs late in COPD and may result in *pulmonary hypertension* and right heart failure (*cor pulmonale*).

Asthma differs markedly from COPD is that there is a greater reversibility spontaneously and with treatment with bronchodilators or steroids (*see* Table 1.1) [2].

Some patients with asthma have progressive irreversible airflow obstruction and therefore have a form of COPD and some patients may have coexistent asthma and COPD. There is still uncertainty as to whether the atopy predisposes to the development of COPD in cigarette smokers (the 'Dutch hypothesis'). Asthma should be regarded as a separate condition from COPD, with different causes, different cellular mechanisms and different responses to treatments. Approximately 10% of patients with COPD may have features of asthma and this is probably accounted for by the coincidence of these common diseases in some patients (*see* Figure 1.1).

Differences between COPD and asthma

	COPD	Asthma
Symptoms	Slowly progressive	Episodic
Signs	Cor pulmonale when severe	Cor pulmonale never seen
Bronchodilator response	<15%	>15%
PEF variability	<15%	>15%
Steroid response	<15%	>15%
Inflammation	Neutrophilic	Eosinophilic

Table 1.1. COPD, chronic obstructive pulmonary disease; PEF, peak expiratory flow.

Overlap between COPD and asthma

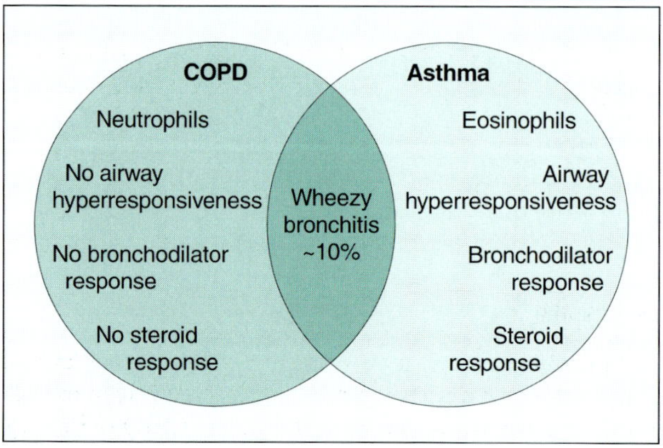

Figure 1.1. Approximately 10% of patients with chronic obstructive pulmonary disease (COPD) have asthma and will share inflammatory features between these diseases. This overlap group may be termed 'wheezy bronchitis'.

The fact that there are different components of COPD has led to attempts to define subgroups with predominant emphysema or intrinsic narrowing of small airways. The terms 'blue bloater' and 'pink puffer' were thought to relate to chronic obstructive bronchitis and emphysema respectively, but it is now apparent that there is enormous overlap in the clinical presentations between these different pathologies and that in most patients these mechanisms coexist; this reflects the fact that cigarette smoking causes both pathologies.

Epidemiology

COPD is a major health problem worldwide and is increasing throughout the world with a high prevalence, high morbidity, high mortality and high cost. It is a leading cause of morbidity and mortality in the adult population. Because the major cause of COPD is cigarette smoking, the epidemiology of COPD largely reflects the demographics of cigarette smoking.

- In the UK, approximately 15–20% of middle aged men and 10% of women report chronic cough and sputum. Most chronic smokers develop mucus hypersecretion (chronic simple bronchitis).
- COPD is diagnosed in approximately 4% of men and 2% of women aged over 45 years in the UK. COPD currently ranks as number six in the global impact of disease scale and is predicted to rise to number three by the year 2020 [3].
- Approximately 6% of deaths in men and 4% in women are due to COPD. In the UK, overall COPD mortality is 200–300/100,000 people aged 45–64 years.
- There are marked differences in mortality and morbidity between countries and these may reflect classification differences. According to the WHO, COPD was the sixth most common cause of death in the world in 1990. In the UK, COPD is the third most common cause of death and in the USA the fourth most common, and is the only common cause of death that is increasing.
- COPD is a very common cause of hospitalization. The mortality of patients who are hospitalized with COPD is almost 15%, which exceeds that of myocardial infarction.
- There have been few changes in the prevalence of COPD over the last 30 years in the UK, in contrast to an increase in asthma. However, there has been a worldwide increase in COPD, reflecting increases in cigarette smoking, especially in developing countries.
- COPD is an important cause of time off work, accounting for 9% of all certified sickness absence in the UK.

Economic and social costs

COPD is a costly public health problem because of its high prevalence. Direct costs are due to hospital admissions and expensive treatments such as long-term oxygen, whereas indirect costs include loss of working capacity and poor quality of life [4].

The amount of disability caused by COPD has been quantified as disability-adjusted life years (DALYs; the sum of years lost because of premature mortality and years of life lived with disability, adjusted for the severity of disability) and was ranked 12th in 1990. The WHO, however, predicted that its rank will rise to five by the year 2020 (*see* Table 1.2) [3].

Leading causes of disability-adjusted life years lost worldwide for 1990 and predicted for 2020

Disease	Rank 1990	Rank 2020
Lower respiratory infections	1	6
Diarrhoeal diseases	2	9
Perinatal conditions	3	11
Unipolar major depression	4	2
Ischaemic heart disease	5	1
Cerebrovascular disease	6	4
Tuberculosis	7	7
Measles	8	25
Road traffic accidents	9	3
Congenital anomalies	10	13
Malaria	11	19
COPD	**12 (2.1% of total)**	**5 (4.1% of total)**

Table 1.2. COPD, chronic obstructive pulmonary disease.

Causes

There are several causative or risk factors involved in COPD (*see* Table 1.3).

Cigarette smoking

Cigarette smoking is by far the most common cause of COPD worldwide, accounting for more than 95% of cases in industrialized countries. Usually there is a smoking history of more than 20 pack-years. Active smoking causes both mucus hypersecretion and chronic airflow obstruction. Cessation of smoking reduces mucus hypersecretion and reduces the rate of decline in lung function. Pipe and cigar smokers have a higher risk for COPD than do non-smokers, although rates are lower than for cigarette smokers. Passive smoking is weakly associated with COPD, mainly via an effect on lung growth during foetal development. Smoking during pregnancy may also be a risk factor for COPD because this may affect lung growth.

Risk factors for COPD	
Environmental factors	**Endogenous factors**
Cigarette smoking Active Passive Maternal	α_1-Antitrypsin deficiency Genetic factors Ethnic factors
Air pollution Outdoor Indoor: biomass fuels	Airway hyperresponsiveness? Atopy
Occupational exposure	Low birth-weight
Dietary factors High salt Low antioxidant vitamins Low unsaturated fatty acids	
Infections	

Table 1.3. COPD, chronic obstructive pulmonary disease.

Air pollution

Air pollution, particularly sulphur dioxide and particulates (black smoke or particulate matter of <10 μm [PM_{10}]), is associated with chronic simple bronchitis and COPD. There may be interactions between cigarette smoking and air pollution. In places where there is heavy air pollution, this may be as important a risk factor as cigarette smoking. Indoor air pollution from biomass fuel that is burned for cooking and heating in poorly ventilated homes may be an important risk factor for COPD in developing countries and this may account for the relatively high rates of disease among women [5].

Occupation

Occupational exposure to fumes, dusts (coal, silica) and solvents may be important and interacts with cigarette smoking. Exposure to cadmium fumes is associated with emphysema.

Infection

Chest infections during the first year of life are associated with COPD in later life [6], but there is little evidence that subsequent chest infections are important. There is some evidence that certain latent virus infections (such as adenovirus) may predispose to the development of COPD [7].

Nutrition

Early nutrition may be important and small-for-date babies have an increased risk of development of COPD in later life [8]. Low dietary intake of antioxidant vitamins (A,

C and E) is also associated with increased risk of COPD [9]. There is some evidence that a diet rich in fish oil is associated with a lower prevalence of COPD.

Atopy

There has been considerable debate about the influence of atopy and airway hyperresponsiveness on the development of COPD. The 'Dutch hypothesis' proposed that atopy and IgE underlie the development of COPD, but there is little evidence for this [10]. COPD itself may result in increased airway responsiveness to histamine or methacholine because of geometric factors related to fixed airway narrowing.

Genetic factors

Genetic factors are probably important and there are several inherited forms of antiprotease deficiency which may predispose to the development of emphysema. The fact that only 10–20% of heavy smokers develop COPD may be largely determined by as yet unidentified genetic factors [11,12]. There appear to be ethnic differences in susceptibility to the effects of cigarette smoking as only 5% of oriental subjects who smoke develop COPD.

It is important to identify the factors that determine why only a small proportion of smokers develop COPD. Thus far this is poorly understood, although it is likely that genetic factors are important [11,12].

- A clearly established genetic risk factor for COPD is the ZZ allele of the α_1-antitrypsin gene, although heterozygotes may be at slightly increased risk. This accounts for more than 1% of cases, however.
- There is an association with a polymorphism of the tumour necrosis factor-alpha (TNF-α) gene (TNF2) that is associated with greater inducibility of TNF-α in a Taiwanese population [13], although this has not been confirmed in Caucasian populations [14].
- There are also weak associations with α_1-antichymotrypsin, α_2-macroglobulin and vitamin D-binding protein.
- A polymorphism in the gene for an enzyme (microsomal epoxide hydrolase) that is responsible for metabolism of reactive epoxide intermediates, which may be generated in tobacco smoke, has been associated with a four- to five-fold increased risk for COPD and emphysema [15], and an association has been confirmed in a large smoking cessation study [16].

Natural history

Patients with COPD usually show an accelerated annual decline in forced expiratory volume in one second (FEV_1), often greater than 50 ml/year, compared with a normal decline of approximately 20 ml/year, although this is variable between patients. The classic studies of Fletcher and Peto [17] established that only 10–20% of cigarette smokers are susceptible. Mortality is related to the amount of cigarettes smoked [18]. Quitting smoking results in a return to the normal rate of decline in lung function and is the only treatment that has so far been able to reduce the rate of decline in patients with COPD (*see* Figure 1.2). These results have been confirmed in the more recent Lung Health Study in the USA [19]. Some patients with COPD have a low baseline FEV_1 and may have a normal rate of decline in lung function but eventually reach a point at which they become symptomatic (*see* Figure 1.3). It can be predicted that these patients would not be susceptible to intervention therapy.

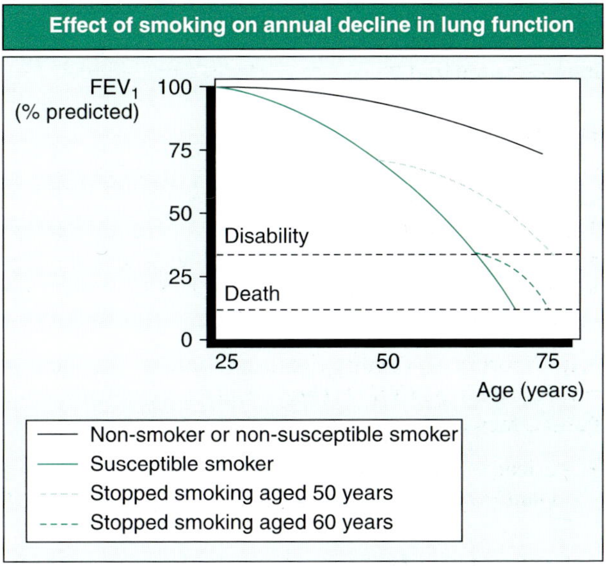

Figure 1.2. Annual decline in airway function showing accelerated decline in susceptible smokers and effects of smoking cessation. Adapted from [17]. © BMJ Publishing Group.

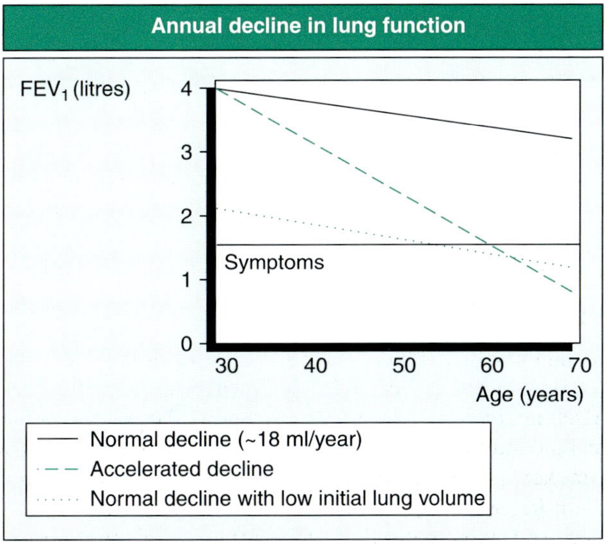

Figure 1.3. Patients with chronic obstructive pulmonary disease may develop airway obstruction from an accelerated rate of decline or a normal rate of decline starting from low initial lung function. FEV_1, forced expiratory volume in one second.

Several factors may influence the natural history of COPD apart from cigarette smoking. Gender does not appear to be important and there is no convincing evidence that males or females are more susceptible to the effects of cigarette smoking. Increased body weight may increase the rate of lung function decline. Airway hyperresponsiveness to histamine and methacholine may increase the rate of decline in lung function, but interpretation is complicated by the fact that a fall in baseline FEV_1 itself increases airway responsiveness purely through geometric mechanisms.

Pathology

- *Chronic bronchitis* is due to hyperplasia of submucosal glands and increased numbers of goblet cells in the epithelium. These changes underlie the mucus hypersecretion found in chronic simple bronchitis.
- *Chronic obstructive bronchitis/bronchiolitis* is associated with structural narrowing of small airways (bronchioles) as a result of chronic inflammatory changes [20,21] (*see* Figure 1.4). These inflammatory changes consist of activated T lymphocytes and macrophages. There are also fibrotic changes that may

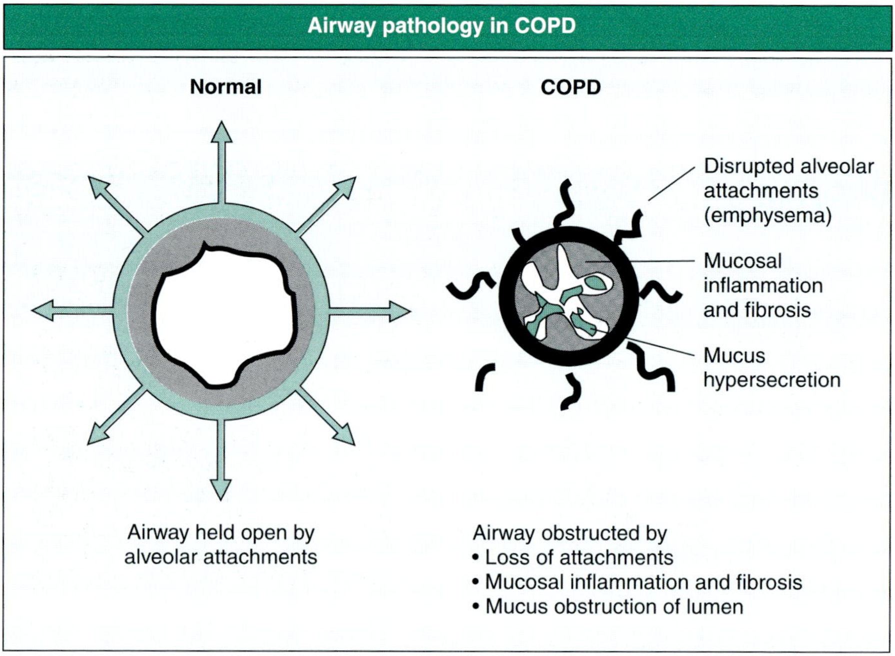

Figure 1.4. The airway in normal subjects is distended by alveolar attachments. In chronic obstructive pulmonary disease (COPD) these attachments are reduced, contributing to airways closure. Peripheral airways are also obstructed by airways inflammation and mucus obstruction.

underlie the irreversible changes that occur in lung function. In larger airways there is evidence of neutrophil inflammation, as judged by increased numbers of neutrophils in bronchoalveolar lavage [22]. Induced sputum exhibits a characteristic increase in the proportion of activated neutrophils which is much greater in patients with COPD than in smokers without obstruction [23–25]. Bronchial biopsies, however, show infiltration with mononuclear cells, $CD4^+$ and particularly cytotoxic ($CD8^+$) T lymphocytes, rather than neutrophils, suggesting that neutrophils may transit rapidly from the circulation into the airway lumen [26]. These changes reflect the inflammatory changes found in small airways [27]. Biopsies and the induced sputum of ex-smokers show a similar inflammatory process, suggesting that inflammation may persist in the airway once it is established [28,29].

- *Emphysema* is due to enzymatic destruction of the alveolar walls. Macrophages and T lymphocytes ($CD8^+$ cells) are prominent at sites of destruction [30,31]. Different patterns of emphysema are observed:
  - *centriacinar,* in which emphysema radiates from the terminal bronchiole;
  - *panacinar,* in which emphysema involves more widespread destruction; and
  - large airspaces together form *bullae.*

Emphysema results in airway obstruction by loss of elastic recoil so that intrapulmonary airways close more readily during expiration.

COPD is associated with both small airway obstruction and emphysema (*see* Figure 1.5), although it is likely that in many patients emphysema is the most important

Peripheral lung pathology of COPD

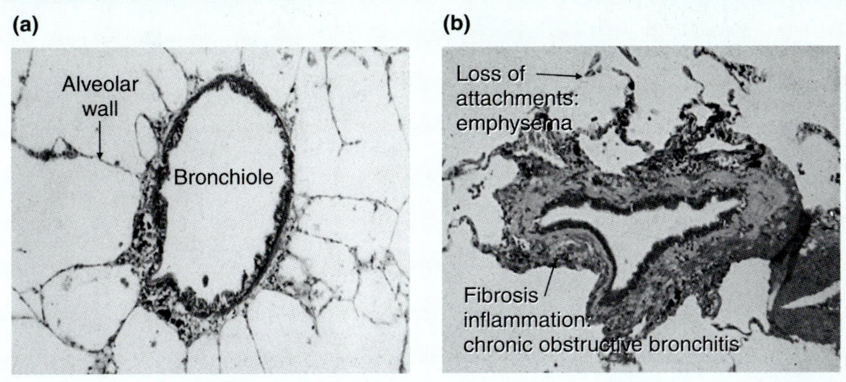

Figure 1.5. **(a)** This panel shows a peripheral airway of a normal person with alveolar attachments intact. **(b)** This panel shows thickening and distortion of a small airway with loss of alveolar attachments. Courtesy of Dr Manuel Cosio (McGill University, Montreal, Canada).

mechanism of chronic airflow obstruction, with the loss of peribronchial alveolar attachments. This results in the loss of driving pressure and airway narrowing with a consequent reduction in FEV_1.

Mechanisms

Mucus hypersecretion

Increased mucus secretion is a result of cigarette smoking or exposure to other inhaled irritants. The mechanism probably involves activation of sensory nerve endings in the airways with reflex (local peptidergic and spinal cholinergic) increase in mucus secretion and direct stimulatory effects of enzymes such as neutrophil elastase and chymase (*see* Figure 1.6). Recent studies suggest that epidermal growth factor (EGF) is a key mediator of mucus hyperplasia and mucus hypersecretion and may be the final common pathway that mediates the effects of many stimuli, including cigarette smoke, on mucus secretion [32]. With time there is hyperplasia of submucosal glands and proliferation of goblet cells under the influence of growth factors such as EGF. Chronic stimulation also leads to up-regulation of mucin (MUC) genes. There are at least eight MUC genes now recognised in humans [33], but it is not yet

Mucus hypersecretion in COPD

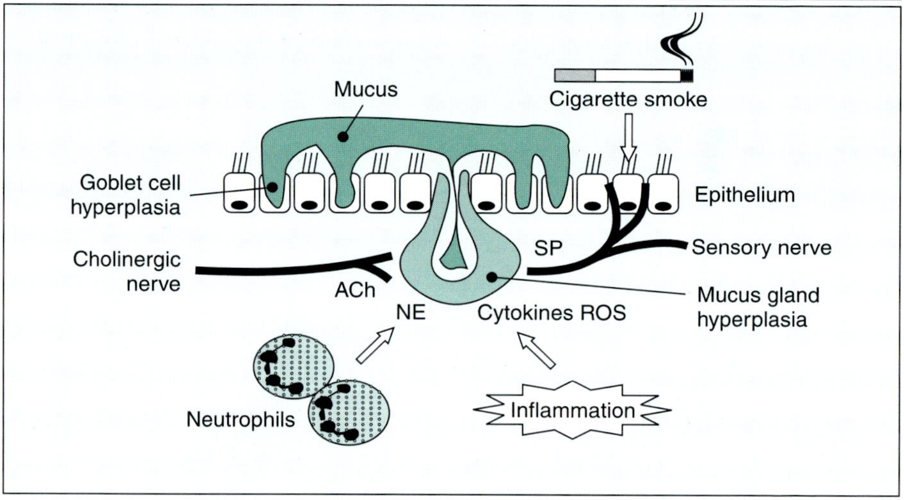

Figure 1.6. Mucus gland secretion may be stimulated via neural mechanisms and the release of acetylcholine (ACh) from cholinergic nerves and of substance P (SP) from sensory nerves. Probably the most important stimulants of mucus secretion are neutrophil elastase (NE) from activated neutrophils and epithelial growth factor (EGF). COPD, chronic obstructive pulmonary disease; ROS, reactive oxygen species.

certain which genes are overexpressed in chronic bronchitis. It was once thought that mucus hypersecretion played no role in airflow obstruction, but recent epidemiological data suggests that mucus hypersecretion is a risk factor for airflow obstruction and it is likely that viscous mucus may contribute to reduced airflow [34].

Small airways obstruction

Obstruction of peripheral airways probably results from a chronic inflammatory process induced by irritants and characterized by neutrophil infiltration, as a result of the release of chemotactic factors, such as interleukin-8 (IL-8) and leukotriene B_4 (LTB_4) from macrophages. This may then result in secretion of fibrogenic mediators, leading to fibrosis of peripheral airways, although this is rarely extensive. Little is known about the mediators involved in peripheral airway inflammation and remodelling.

Protease-antiprotease imbalance

Emphysema is due to an imbalance between proteases (that digest elastin and other structural proteins in the alveolar wall) and antiproteases, that protect against this attack (*see* Figure 1.7) [35].

Several proteases are likely to be involved in lung parenchymal destruction:

- *Neutrophil elastase*, a neutral serine protease, is a major constituent of lung elastolytic activity and also potently stimulates mucus secretion. In addition, neutrophil elastase induces IL-8 release from epithelial cells and therefore may perpetuate the inflammatory state. Although neutrophil elastase is likely to be the major mechanism mediating elastolysis in patients with alpha-1-antitrypsin

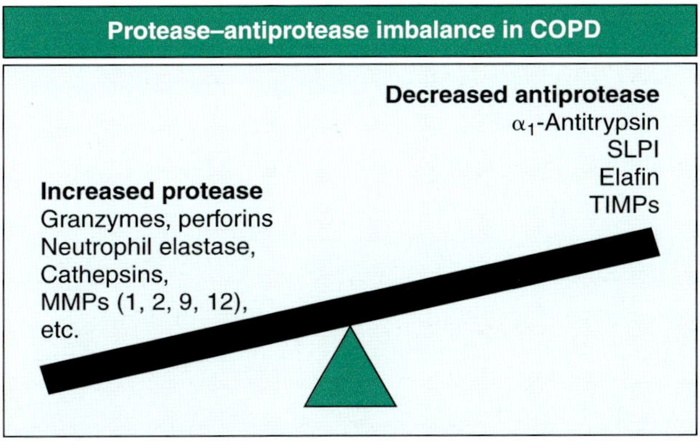

Figure 1.7. In chronic obstructive pulmonary disease (COPD) the balance appears to be tipped in favour of increased proteolysis, either because of an increase in proteases, including neutrophil elastase, cathepsins and matrix metalloproteinases (MMP), or a deficiency in antiproteases, which may include α_1-antitrypsin, elafin, secretory leukoprotease inhibitor (SLPI) and tissue inhibitors of matrix metalloproteinases (TIMPs).

(α_1-AT) deficiency, it may well not be the major elastolytic enzyme in smoking-related COPD, and it is important to consider other enzymes as targets for inhibition.

- *Proteinase 3* is another neutral serine protease in neutrophils and may contribute to the elastolytic activity of these cells.
- *Cathepsin G* is a cysteine protease in neutrophils that also has elastolytic activity. Cathepsins B, L and S are also released from macrophages.
- *Matrix metalloproteinases* (MMP) are a group of over 20 closely related endopeptidases that are capable of degrading all of the components of the extracellular matrix of lung parenchyma, including elastin, collagen, proteoglycans, laminin and fibronectin. They are produced by neutrophils, alveolar macrophages and airway epithelial cells [36]. Increased levels of collagenase (MMP-1) and gelatinase B (MMP-9) have been detected in bronchoalveolar lavage fluid of patients with emphysema [37]. Lavaged macrophages from patients with emphysema express more MMP-9 and MMP-1 than do cells from control individuals, suggesting that these cells, rather than neutrophils, may be the major cellular source [38]. Alveolar macrophages also express a unique MMP, macrophage metalloelastase (MMP-12) [39]. MMP-12 knock-out mice do not develop emphysema and do not show the expected increases in lung macrophages after long-term exposure to cigarette smoke [40]. MMP-12 does not appear to play a major role in humans and MMP-9 is probably a major elastolytic enzyme in emphysema.

Counterbalancing these proteases is a range of *antiproteases*:

- *α_1-Antitrypsin* (α_1-AT, also known as α_1-protease inhibitor) is the major antiprotease in lung parenchyma. It is mainly derived from plasma and synthesized in the liver. Inheritance of homozygous α_1-AT deficiency may result in severe emphysema, particularly in cigarette smokers, but this genetic disease accounts for less than 1% of cases of COPD. α_1-AT is the major protease that counteracts the effects of neutrophil elastase, but it is not the only antiprotease.
- *α_1-Antichymotrypsin* is also present in the lungs and heterozygous individuals that have lower than normal levels have an increased risk of COPD.
- *Secretory leukocyte protease inhibitor* (SLPI) is the most important protective mechanism in the airways. It is derived from airway epithelial cells and provides a local protective mechanism.
- *Tissue inhibitors of metalloproteinases* (TIMPs) counteract the effect of matrix metalloproteinases.

Oxidative stress

There is considerable evidence that oxidative stress is increased in patients with COPD and that reactive oxygen species contribute to its pathophysiology [41,42]. Oxidants are present in cigarette smoke (each puff of cigarette smoke contains 10^{17} free radicals) and are produced endogenously by activated inflammatory cells, including neutrophils and alveolar macrophages. Increased production of endogenous oxidants is demonstrated by the increased levels of hydrogen peroxide (H_2O_2) in expired condensates from patients with COPD, particularly during exacerbations [43]. There is also an increase in concentrations of ethane in exhaled air and in 8-isoprostane in exhaled breath condensate from COPD patients, indicating increased oxidative stress, which is related to disease severity [44,45].

Oxidants may contribute to the pathophysiology of COPD in several ways, including damage of serum protease inhibitors, potentiation of elastase activity and increased mucus secretion. In addition oxidants activate the transcription factor nuclear factor-κB (NF-κB), which orchestrates the transcription of many inflammatory genes, including IL-8, inducible nitric oxide synthase and inducible cyclooxygenase (COX-2) (*see* Figure 1.8). Oxidative stress also leads to the formation of isoprostanes by direct oxidation of

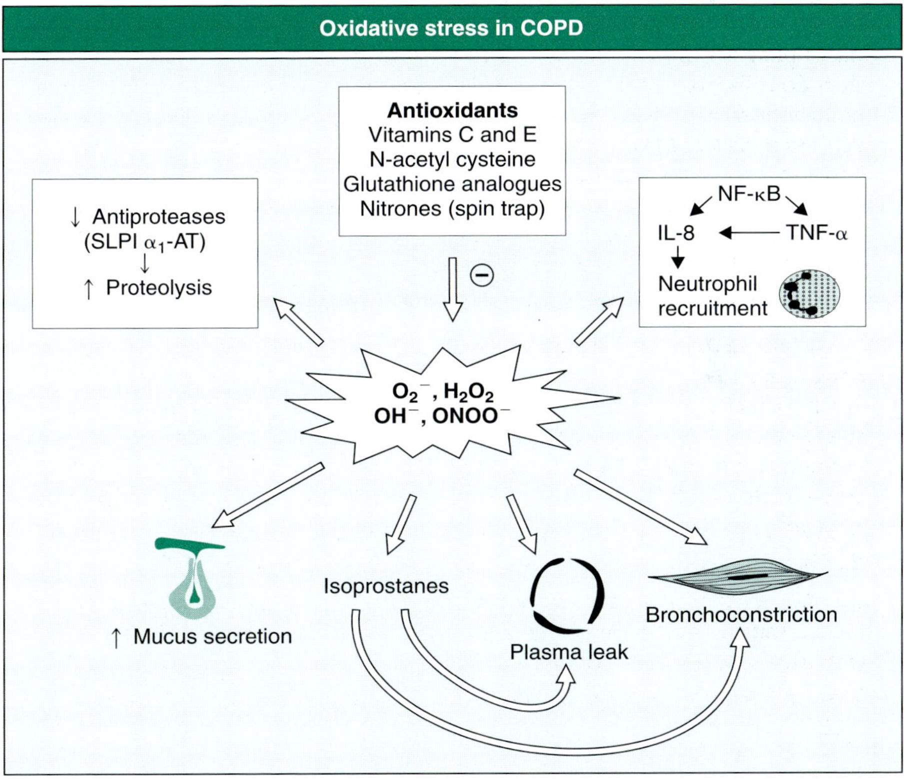

Figure 1.8. Reactive oxygen species from cigarette smoke or from inflammatory cells result in several damaging effects in chronic obstructive pulmonary disease (COPD), including decreased antiprotease defences, activation of nuclear factor-κB (NF-κB) resulting in increased secretion of the cytokines interleukin-8 (IL-8) and tumour necrosis factor-alpha (TNF-α), increased production of isoprostanes and direct effects on airway functions. SLPI, secretory leukoprotease inhibitor; AT, antitrypsin.

arachidonic acid. Isoprostanes are increased in COPD [45,46] and may have several effects on airway function, including bronchoconstriction, increased plasma leakage and mucus hypersecretion.

Bronchiolitis versus emphysema

There is debate about whether the airflow obstruction in COPD is primarily due to obstruction of the lumen of small airways as a result of bronchiolitis [47], or whether it is due to loss of elasticity and closure of small airways as a result of parenchymal destruction. Loss of lung elasticity may occur in COPD even in the absence of emphysema and it is likely that this may be an important contributor to airway obstruction in all patients with COPD. The extent to which peripheral airway obstruction as a result of fibrosis and lumenal obstruction with mucus contributes to airflow limitation probably varies from patient to patient, but it is likely that both mechanisms contribute to a variable extent in most patients, because cigarette smoking causes both abnormalities.

Cellular mechanisms

The mechanisms of inflammation in COPD are not yet certain. Cigarette smoking and other inhaled irritants may initiate an inflammatory response in the peripheral airways and lung parenchyma. It is likely that neutrophil chemotactic factors are released from activated macrophages and possibly from epithelial cells and $CD8^+$ (cytotoxic) T lymphocytes (*see* Figure 1.9). Macrophages may play an important role in driving the inflammatory process in COPD and may release neutrophil chemotactic factors as well as proteolytic enzymes. Macrophages may be activated by cigarette smoke and other inhaled irritants. Macrophage numbers are increased by five- to 10-fold in bronchoalveolar lavage of patients with COPD and are concentrated in the centriacinar zones where emphysema is most marked. Furthermore, the numbers of macrophages and T lymphocytes, but not the numbers of neutrophils, in the alveolar wall correlate with the amount of parenchymal destruction [30]. Macrophages may be responsible for the continued proteolytic activity in the lungs of patients with emphysema and release increased amounts of inflammatory mediators and proteinases in COPD. The role of cytotoxic T cells is still uncertain, but they may be important in the development of emphysema by inducing apoptosis of type 1 alveolar cells.

There are striking differences in inflammation between asthma and COPD, with differences in inflammatory cells, mediators, inflammatory effects and location of the inflammatory process (*see* Table 1.4 and Figure 1.10). In some situations, however, the distinctions are less clear; in severe asthma there is also an increase in neutrophils [48], whereas in exacerbations of COPD there may be an increase in eosinophils [49].

Inflammatory mediators

Several inflammatory mediators are involved in the pathophysiology of COPD (*see* Figure 1.11) as follows.

Inflammatory mechanisms in COPD

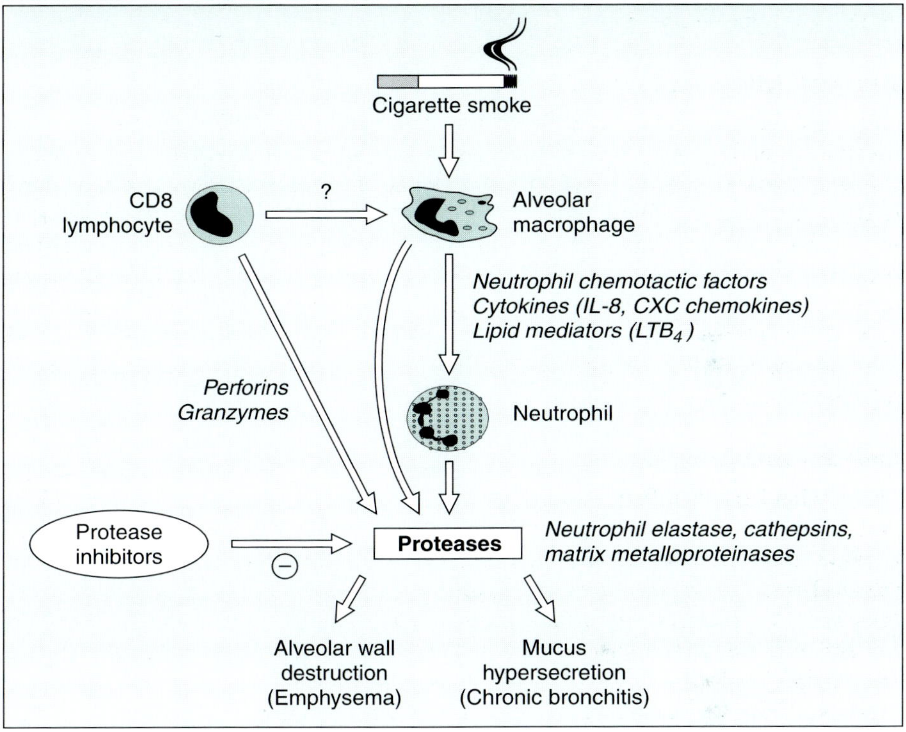

Figure 1.9. Cigarette smoke (and other irritants) activate macrophages in the respiratory tract that release neutrophil chemotactic factors, including interleukin-8 (IL-8) and leukotriene B_4 (LTB_4). These cells then release proteases that break down connective tissue in the lung parenchyma, resulting in emphysema, and also stimulate mucus hypersecretion. These enzymes are normally counteracted by protease inhibitors, including α_1-antitrypsin, secretory leukoprotease inhibitor (SLPI) and tissue inhibitor of matrix metalloproteinases (TIMP). Cytotoxic T cells ($CD8^+$) may also be involved in the inflammatory cascade. COPD, chronic obstructive pulmonary disease.

- *LTB_4*: there are increased amounts of LTB_4, a potent chemoattractant of neutrophils, in the sputum of patients with COPD [50]. Alveolar macrophages from patients with α_1-antitrypsin deficiency secrete greater amounts of LTB_4 [51]. IL-8 is another chemoattractant for neutrophils and is present in high concentrations in the induced sputum of patients with COPD (*see* Figure 1.12) [23,52].
- *Chemokines*: IL-8 may be secreted by macrophages, neutrophils and by airway epithelial cells [53]. IL-8 may be important in the neutrophil inflammation found

Differences between inflammation in COPD and in asthma		
Inflammation	**COPD**	**Asthma**
Inflammatory cells		Mast cells
	Neutrophils	Eosinophils
	$CD8^+$ cells	$CD4^+$ cells
	Macrophages ++	Macrophages +
Inflammatory mediators	LTB_4	LTD_4, histamine
	TNF-α	IL-4, IL-5, IL-13
	IL-8, GRO-α	Eotaxin, RANTES
	Oxidative stress +++	Oxidative stress +
Inflammatory effects	Peripheral airways	All airways
	Airway hyperresponsiveness ±	Airway hyperresponsiveness +++
	Epithelial metaplasia	Epithelial shedding
	Fibrosis ++	Fibrosis +
	Parenchymal destruction	No parenchymal involvement
	Mucus secretion +++	Mucus secretion +
Response to corticosteroids	±	+++

Table 1.4. COPD, chronic obstructive pulmonary disease; LT, leukotriene; TNF, tumour necrosis factor; IL, interleukin; GRO, growth-related oncogene; RANTES, regulated on activation normal T-cell expressed and secreted.

in induced sputum of patients with COPD and is correlated with the number of neutrophils, which in turn correlate with the degree of airflow obstruction (*see* Figure 1.11). Other chemokines may also be important in COPD; growth related oncogene-α (GRO-α) which is elevated in COPD, is chemotactic for monocytes as well as neutrophils and may therefore contribute to the increased numbers of macrophages that are derived from blood monocytes in COPD.

- *TNF-α*: also present in high concentration in the sputum of COPD patients, TNF-α may activate the transcription of NF-κB, which switches on the transcription of the IL-8 gene [54] (*see* Figure 1.13).
- *Endothelin*: endothelin-1 (ET-1) levels are increased in the sputum of patients with COPD and may be important in pulmonary vascular remodelling in severe disease [55].
- *T cell mediators*: the role of T lymphocytes in COPD is unknown. The predominance of $CD8^+$ cells (suppressor T cells) may contribute to

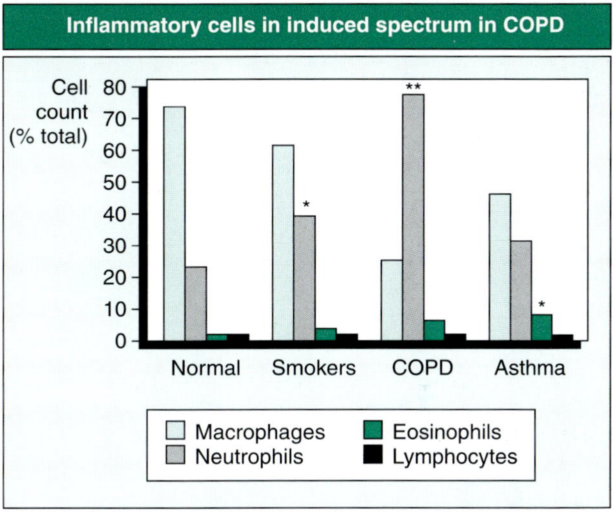

Figure 1.10. There are increased numbers of neutrophils in induced sputum of patients with chronic obstructive pulmonary disease (COPD), whereas eosinophils are increased in asthma. Normal cigarette smokers also have an increase in neutrophils, but this is less than that seen in patients with COPD who have a similar smoking history. Patient group sizes: normal (n=16); smokers (n=12); COPD (n=14); asthma (n=22). *$p<0.05$; **$p<0.01$. Adapted from [23]. © American Lung Association.

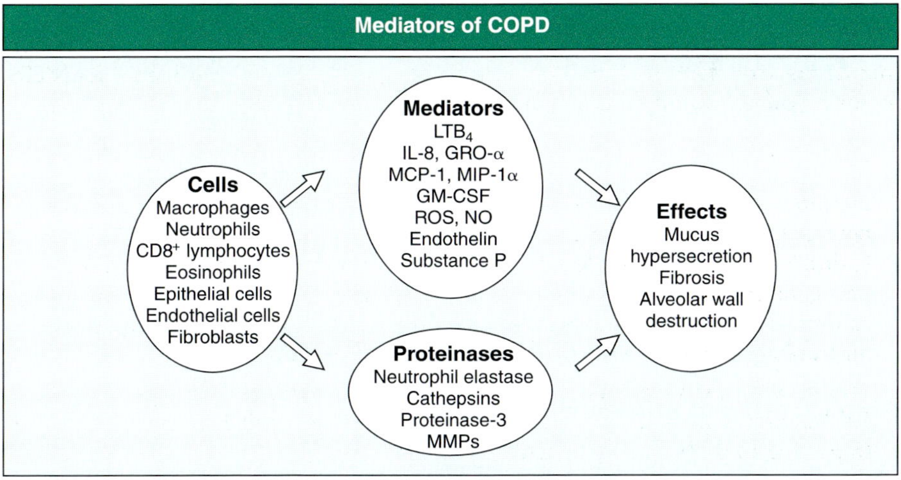

Figure 1.11. Many mediators and proteases are released in chronic obstructive pulmonary disease (COPD). LTB_4, leukotriene B_4, IL, interleukin; GRO, growth related oncogene; MCP, monocyte chemotactic protein; MIP, monocyte inflammatory protein; GM-CSF, granulocyte-macrophage colony stimulating factor; ROS, reactive oxygen species; NO, nitric oxide; MMP, matrix metalloproteinases.

Increased cytokine production in COPD

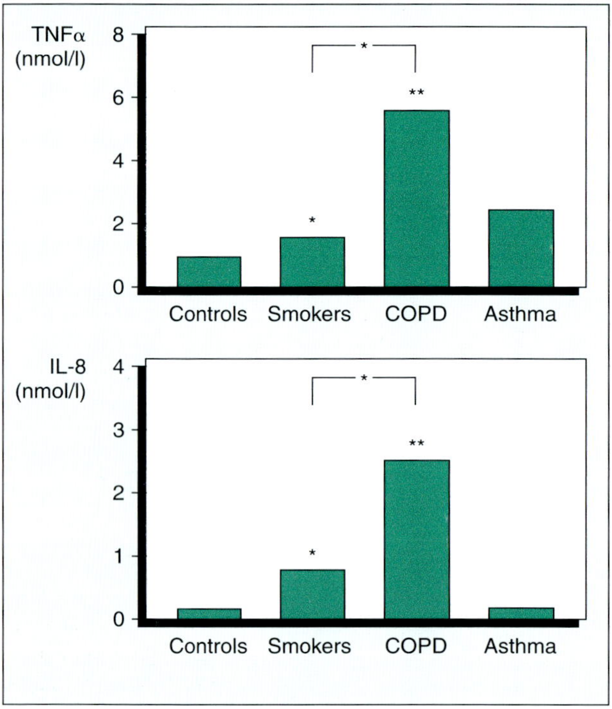

Figure 1.12. There are increased levels of tumour necrosis factor-alpha (TNF-α) and interleukin-8 (IL-8) in induced sputum of patients with chronic obstructive pulmonary disease (COPD; n=14) compared with normal subjects (n=16), cigarette smokers without airway obstruction (n=12) and patients with asthma (n=22). The patients with COPD had a mean age of 62.5±3.2 years and forced expiratory volume in one second (FEV_1) of 34.6±4% of predicted value. Adapted from [23]. © American Lung Association.

pathophysiology via the release of enzymes, such as granzymes and perforins that may induce apoptosis in parenchymal cells [56,57].

Amplification of inflammation

Inflammation in normal smokers is very similar in terms of inflammatory cells, mediators and proteases compared with patients with COPD, but is less pronounced. This suggests that the inflammation in COPD lungs represents an exaggeration of the normal inflammatory response to irritants, such as cigarette smoke (*see* Figure 1.14) [20]. The mechanisms for this amplification are not yet certain, but may be determined by genetic factors, by a latent virus (such as adenovirus), by oxidative stress or by some molecular amplification process that is not yet understood.

Effect of cigarette smoking on cytokine release

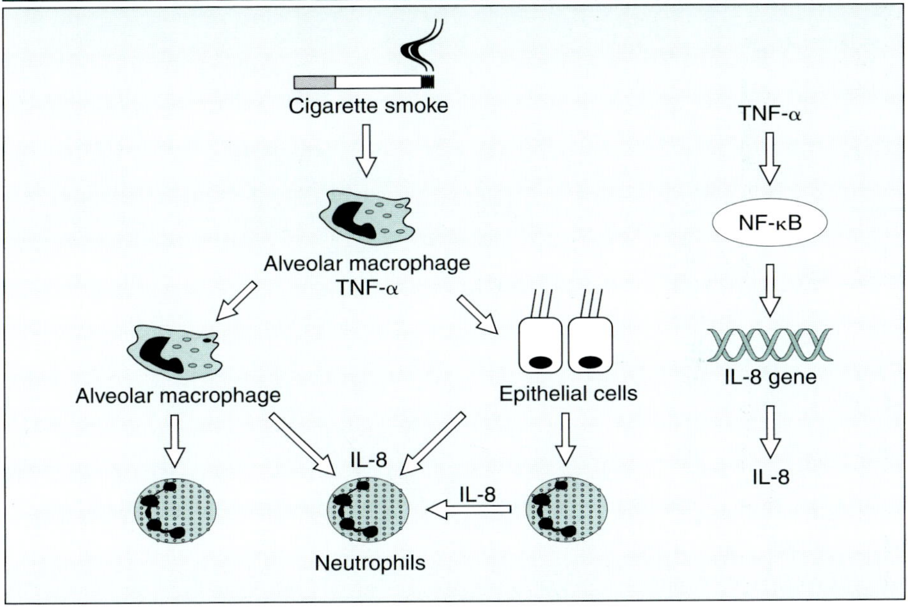

Figure 1.13. Cigarette smoke activates macrophages to release tumour necrosis factor-alpha (TNF-α), which releases interleukin-8 (IL-8) via activation of the transcription factor nuclear factor-κB (NF-κB). IL-8 attracts neutrophils, which themselves secrete IL-8 to perpetuate the response.

Vascular pathology

Chronic hypoxia results in widespread pulmonary vasoconstriction and pulmonary hypertension. This leads to remodelling of the pulmonary circulation. These changes include:

- extension of vascular smooth muscle to vessels that normally lack muscle;
- intimal hyperplasia; and
- fibrosis and obliteration of some vessels.

These changes may lead to right heart failure (cor pulmonale) in some patients (*see* Figure 1.15).

The mechanisms of remodelling are not yet understood and it is likely that several growth factors, including vascular endothelial growth factor and fibroblast growth factor, may be involved. Endothelin-1 (ET-1) is strongly expressed in pulmonary vascular endothelium of patients with pulmonary hypertension secondary to chronic hypoxia [58]. Urinary ET-1 excretion is increased in patients with COPD [59] and sputum ET-1 levels are increased in exacerbations [55]. ET-1, acting mainly via ETA

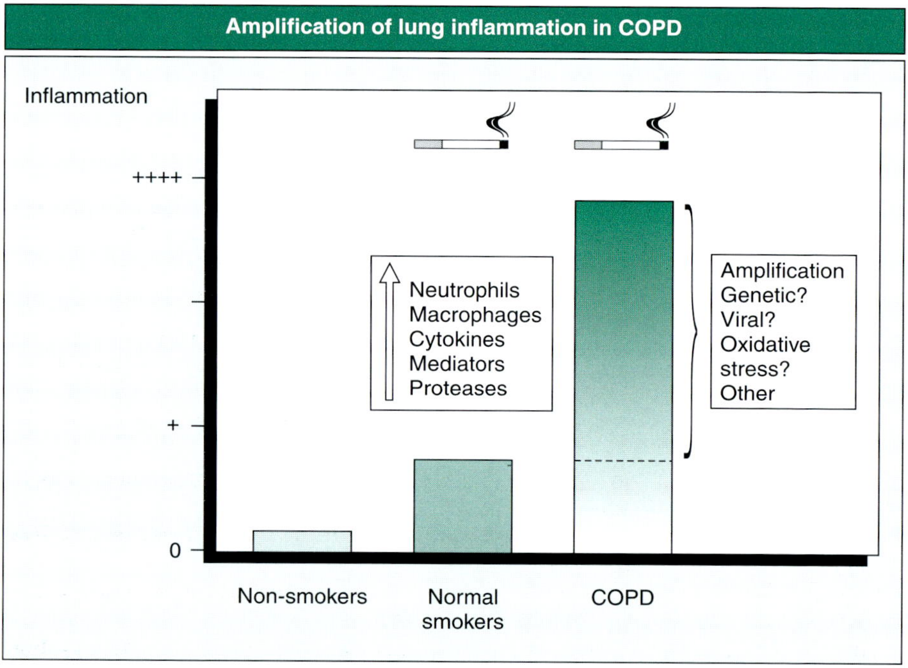

Figure 1.14. Normal smokers have an inflammatory response, but this appears to be amplified in patients with chronic obstructive pulmonary disease (COPD). The molecular mechanisms of this amplification are currently unknown.

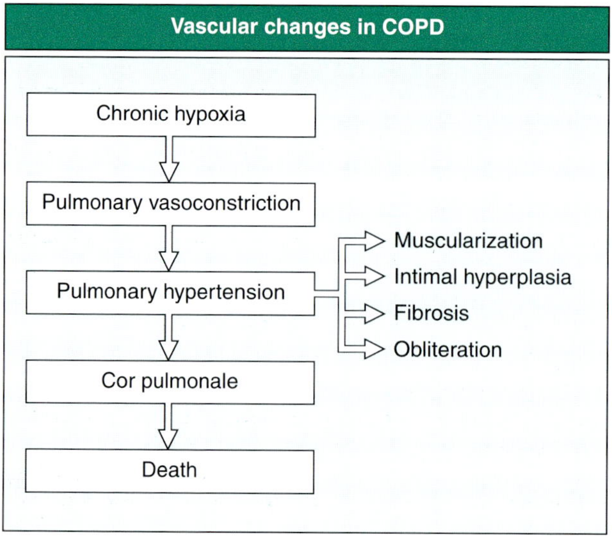

Figure 1.15. Chronic hypoxia results in hypoxic pulmonary vasoconstriction and over time leads to structural changes, resulting in secondary pulmonary hypertension. Over time this may lead to right heart failure (cor pulmonale), which has a poor prognosis. COPD, chronic obstructive pulmonary disease.

receptors, induces fibrosis and hyperplasia of pulmonary vascular smooth muscle, implying a role in the pulmonary hypertension secondary to COPD.

References

1. Pauwels RA, Buist AS, Calverley PMA *et al.* **Global strategy for the diagnosis, management and prevention of chronic obstructive pulmonary disease.** *Am J Respir Crit Care Med* 2001; **163**:1256–1276.

2. Barnes PJ. **Mechanisms in COPD: differences from asthma.** *Chest* 2000; **117**(Suppl):10S–14S.

3. Lopez AD, Murray CC. **The global burden of disease, 1990–2020.** *Nat Med* 1998; **4**:1241–1243.

4. Sullivan SD, Ramsey SD, Lee TA. **The economic burden of COPD.** *Chest* 2000; **117**(Suppl):5S–9S.

5. Dennis RJ, Maldonado D, Norman S *et al.* **Woodsmoke exposure and risk for obstructive airways disease among women.** *Chest* 1996; **109**:115–119.

6. Strachan DP, Seagroatt V, Cook DG. **Chest illness in infancy and chronic respiratory disease in later life: an analysis by month of birth.** *Int J Epidemiol* 1994; **23**:1060–1068.

7. Matsuse T, Hayashi S, Kuwano K *et al.* **Latent adenoviral infection in the pathogenesis of chronic airways obstruction.** *Am Rev Respir Dis* 1992; **146**:177–184.

8. Barker DJP, Osmond C, Law CM. **The intrauterine and early postnatal origins of cardiovascular disease and chronic bronchitis.** *J Epidemiol Community Health* 1989; **43**:237–240.

9. Britton JR, Pavord ID, Richards KA *et al.* **Dietary antioxidant vitamin intake and lung function in the general population.** *Am J Respir Crit Care Med* 1995; **151**:1383–1387.

10. Pride N. **Smoking, allergy and airways obstruction: revival of the 'Dutch hypothesis'.** *Clin Allergy* 1986; **16**:3–6.

11. Sandiford AJ, Weir TD, Pare PD. **Genetic risk factors for chronic obstructive pulmonary disease.** *Eur Respir J* 1997; **10**:1380–1391.

12. Barnes PJ. **Molecular genetics of chronic obstructive pulmonary disease.** *Thorax* 1999; **54**:245–252.

13. Huang SL, Su CH, Chang SC. **Tumor necrosis factor-alpha gene polymorphism in chronic bronchitis.** *Am J Respir Crit Care Med* 1997; **156**:1436–1439.

14. Higham MA, Pride NB, Alikhan A *et al.* **Tumour necrosis factor-α gene promoter polymorphism in chronic obstructive pulmonary disease.** *Eur Respir J* 2000; **15**:281–284.

15. Smith CAD, Harrison DJ. **Association between polymorphism in gene for microsomal epoxide hydrolase and susceptibility to emphysema.** *Lancet* 1997; **350**:630–633.

16. Sandford AJ, Chagani T, Weir TD *et al.* **Susceptibility genes for rapid decline of lung function in the lung health study.** *Am J Respir Crit Care Med* 2001; **163**:469–473.

17. Fletcher C, Peto R. **The natural history of chronic airflow obstruction.** *BMJ* 1977; **1**:1645–1648.

18. Doll R, Peto R, Wheatley K *et al.* **Mortality in relation to smoking: 40 years' observations on male British doctors.** *BMJ* 1994; **309**:901–911.

19. Anthonisen NR, Connett JE, Kiley JP *et al.* **Effects of smoking intervention and the use of an inhaled anticholinergic bronchodilator on the rate of decline of FEV_1.** *JAMA* 1994; **272**:1497–1505.

20. Barnes PJ. **Chronic obstructive pulmonary disease.** *N Engl J Med* 2000; **343**:269–280.

21. Turato G, Zuin R, Saetta M. **Pathogenesis and pathology of COPD.** *Respiration* 2001; **68**:117–128.

22. Thompson PB, Daughton D, Robbins GA *et al.* **Intramural airway inflammation in chronic bronchitis. Characterization and correlation with clinical parameters.** *Am Rev Respir Dis* 1989; **140**:1527–1537.

23. Keatings VM, Collins PD, Scott DM *et al.* **Differences in interleukin-8 and tumor necrosis factor-alpha in induced sputum from patients with chronic obstructive pulmonary disease or asthma.** *Am J Respir Crit Care Med* 1996; **153**:530–534.

24. Keatings VM, Barnes PJ. **Granulocyte activation markers in induced sputum: comparison between chronic obstructive pulmonary disease, asthma and normal subjects.** *Am J Respir Crit Care Med* 1997; **155**:449–453.

25. Peleman RA, Rytila PH, Kips JC *et al.* **The cellular composition of induced sputum in chronic obstructive pulmonary disease.** *Eur Respir J* 1999; **13**:839–843.

26. Jeffery PK. **Structural and inflammatory changes in COPD: a comparison with asthma.** *Thorax* 1998; **53**:129–36.

27. Saetta M, Turato G, Baraldo S *et al.* **Goblet cell hyperplasia and epithelial inflammation in peripheral airways of smokers with both symptoms of chronic bronchitis and chronic airflow limitation.** *Am J Respir Crit Care Med* 2000; **161**:1016–1021.

28. Turato G, Di Stefano A, Maestrelli P *et al.* **Effect of smoking cessation on airway inflammation in chronic bronchitis.** *Am J Respir Crit Care Med* 1995; **152**:1262–1267.

29. Rutgers SR, Postma DS, ten Hacken NH *et al.* **Ongoing airway inflammation in patients with COPD who do not currently smoke.** *Thorax* 2000; **55**:12–18.

30. Finkelstein R, Fraser RS, Ghezzo H *et al.* **Alveolar inflammation and its relation to emphysema in smokers.** *Am J Respir Crit Care Med* 1995; **152**:1666–1672.

31. Saetta M, Di Stefano A, Turato G *et al.* **$CD8^+$ T-lymphocytes in peripheral airways of smokers with chronic obstructive pulmonary disease.** *Am J Respir Crit Care Med* 1998; **157**:822–826.

32. Takeyama K, Dabbagh K, Lee HM *et al.* **Epidermal growth factor system regulates mucin production in airways.** *Proc Natl Acad Sci USA* 1999; **96**:3081–3086.

33. Reid CJ, Gould S, Harris A. **Developmental expression of mucin genes in the human respiratory tract.** *Am J Respir Cell Mol Biol* 1997; **17**:592–598.

34. Vestbo J, Prescott E, Lange P. **Association of chronic mucus hypersecretion with FEV_1 decline and chronic obstructive pulmonary disease morbidity. Copenhagen City Heart Study Group.** *Am J Respir Crit Care Med* 1996; **153**:1530–1535.

35. Stockley RA. **The role of proteinases in the pathogenesis of chronic bronchitis.** *Am J Respir Crit Care Med* 1994; **150**(Suppl):S109–S113.

36. Shapiro SD. **Elastolytic metalloproteinases produced by human mononuclear phagocytes. Potential roles in destructive lung disease.** *Am J Respir Crit Care Med* 1994; **150**(Suppl): S160–S164.

37. Finlay GA, Russell KJ, McMahon KJ *et al.* **Elevated levels of matrix metalloproteinases in bronchoalveolar lavage fluid of emphysematous patients.** *Thorax* 1997; **52**:502–506.

38. Finlay GA, O'Driscoll LR, Russell KJ *et al.* **Matrix metalloproteinase expression and production by alveolar macrophages in emphysema.** *Am J Respir Crit Care Med* 1997; **156**:240–247.

39. Shapiro SG, Kobayashi DK, Ley TJ. **Cloning and characterization of a unique elastolytic metalloproteinase produced by human alveolar macrophages.** *J Biol Chem* 1993; **268**:23824–23829.

40. Hautamaki RD, Kobayashi DK, Senior RM *et al.* **Requirement for macrophage metalloelastase for cigarette smoke-induced emphysema in mice.** *Science* 1997; **277**:2002–2004.

41. Repine JE, Bast A, Lankhorst I. **Oxidative stress in chronic obstructive pulmonary disease.** *Am J Respir Crit Care Med* 1997; **156**:341–357.

42. Macnee W. **Oxidants/antioxidants and COPD.** *Chest* 2000; **117**(Suppl):303S–317S.

43. Dekhuijzen PNR, Aben KHH, Dekker I *et al.* **Increased exhalation of hydrogen peroxide in patients with stable and unstable chronic obstructive pulmonary disease.** *Am J Respir Crit Care Med* 1996; **154**:813–816.

44. Paredi P, Kharitonov SA, Leak D *et al.* **Exhaled ethane, a marker of lipid peroxidation, is elevated in chronic obstructive pulmonary disease.** *Am J Respir Crit Care Med* 2000; **162**:369–373.

45. Montuschi P, Collins JV, Ciabattoni G *et al.* **Exhaled 8-isoprostane as an *in vivo* biomarker of lung oxidative stress in patients with COPD and healthy smokers.** *Am J Respir Crit Care Med* 2000; **162**:1175–1177.

46. Pratico D, Basili S, Vieri M *et al.* **Chronic obstructive pulmonary disease is associated with an increase in urinary levels of isoprostane F2a-III, an index of oxidant stress.** *Am J Respir Crit Care Med* 1998; **158**:1709–1714.

47. Gelb AF, Hogg JC, Muller NL *et al.* **Contribution of emphysema and small airways in COPD.** *Chest* 1996; **109**: 353–359.

48. Jatakanon A, Uasaf C, Maziak W *et al.* **Neutrophilic inflammation in severe persistent asthma.** *Am J Respir Crit Care Med* 1999; **160**:1532–1539.

49. Saetta M, Distefano A, Maestrelli P *et al.* **Airway eosinophilia in chronic bronchitis during exacerbations.** *Am J Respir Crit Care Med* 1994; **150**:1646–1652.

50. Hill AT, Bayley D, Stockley RA. **The interrelationship of sputum inflammatory markers in patients with chronic bronchitis.** *Am J Respir Crit Care Med* 1999; **160**:893–898.

51. Hubbard RC, Fells G, Gadek J *et al.* **Neutrophil accumulation in the lung in α1-antitrypsin deficiency. Spontaneous release of leukotriene B_4 by alveolar macrophages.** *J Clin Invest* 1991; **88**:891–897.

52. Yamamoto C, Yoneda T, Yoshikawa M *et al.* **Airway inflammation in COPD assessed by sputum levels of interleukin-8.** *Chest* 1997; **112**:505–510.

53. Kwon OJ, Au BT, Collins PD *et al.* **Tumor necrosis factor-induced interleukin 8 expression in cultured human epithelial cells.** *Am J Physiol* 1994; **11**:L398–L405.

54. Barnes PJ, Karin M. **Nuclear factor-κB: a pivotal transcription factor in chronic inflammatory diseases.** *N Engl J Med* 1997; **336**:1066–1071.

55. Roland M, Bhowmik A, Sapsford RJ *et al.* **Sputum and plasma endothelin-1 levels in exacerbations of chronic obstructive pulmonary disease.** *Thorax* 2001; **56**:30–35.

56. Liu AN, Mohammed AZ, Rice WR *et al.* **Perforin-independent CD8(+) T-cell-mediated cytotoxicity of alveolar epithelial cells is preferentially mediated by tumor necrosis factor-alpha: relative insensitivity to Fas ligand.** *Am J Respir Cell Mol Biol* 1999; **20**:849–858.

57. Majo J, Ghezzo H, Cosio MG. **Lymphocyte population and apoptosis in the lungs of smokers and their relation to emphysema.** *Eur Respir J* 2001; **17**:946–953.

58. Giaid A, Yanagisawa M, Langleben D *et al.* **Expression of endothelin-l in the lungs of patients with pulmonary hypertension.** *N Engl J Med* 1993; **328**:1732–1739.

59. Sofia M, Mormile M, Faraone S *et al.* **Increased 24-hour endothelin-1 urinary excretion in patients with chronic obstructive pulmonary disease.** *Respiration* 1994; **61**:263–268.

Chapter 2

Clinical features

The term COPD in adults implies the common type of chronic lung disease with airways obstruction usually related to heavy smoking and excluding other generalized conditions such as asthma and obliterative bronchiolitis or localized conditions such as bronchiectasis. The patient may, of course, have more than one lung disease at the same time; for example, COPD and carcinoma of the lung may well coexist in a heavy smoker, and some patients may have COPD and asthma.

The clinical features of COPD are usually straightforward and care should be taken to evaluate those features of the illness that are not typical.

Symptoms

The symptoms of COPD are slowly progressive over many years, in contrast to the episodic and variable symptoms of asthma. Patients have usually lost a considerable amount of their lung volume by the time they present to a doctor, with FEV_1 values below 50%. There is usually a history of heavy smoking for many years, often more than 25 pack years (one pack year equals 20 cigarettes daily for one year).

Cough and sputum

- Cough and sputum production for many years, often worse in the winter months.
- Cough often present only on waking at first but rarely disturbs sleep.
- Later, cough occurs throughout the day.
- Sputum usually mucoid — becomes purulent with exacerbation of disease and not usually excessive (<1 eggcupful/day).
- Cough syncope may occur after prolonged bouts of coughing.

Breathlessness

- Insidious onset on exertion with compensatory behaviour to reduce symptoms.
- Related to changes in end-expiratory volume during exercise [1].
- Later leads to reliance on accessory muscles of respiration.
- Some develop increasingly severe exacerbations of disease leading to chronic respiratory failure and heart failure — 'blue bloater' type of COPD.
- Others have little or no sputum or hypoxia at rest but breathlessness and wheezing is severe and emphysema is prominent — 'pink puffer' type of COPD. These patients are commonly underweight.
- Most patients with COPD present with a mixed pattern rather than the 'blue bloater' or 'pink puffer' extremes.

Other symptoms

- *Wheezing* may occur during exacerbations and during periods of breathlessness.
- *Chest pains* are common and may be due to concomitant ischaemic heart disease or strain on intercostal muscles.
- *Ankle swelling* may occur when there is cor pulmonale.
- *Anorexia and weight loss* often occur in advanced disease, but the mechanism is uncertain. It may be due to increased work of breathing or increased production of TNF-α [2]. Recent weight loss should prompt a search for an underlying carcinoma.
- *Skeletal muscle wasting* occurs in some patients, usually with advanced COPD. This appears to be due to apoptosis of skeletal muscles that may result from increased systemic production of TNF-α [3].
- *Depression and malaise* are common features of severe COPD and may reflect increased systemic production of cytokines [4].

Symptoms not typical of COPD

- Haemoptysis — can occur just due to COPD but its appearance in such a patient suggests the possibility of malignancy, which must be carefully investigated.
- Seasonal exacerbations in spring or summer are more likely in asthma.
- Excellent response to bronchodilators or steroids with definite symptom-free intervals is suggestive of asthma, not COPD.
- Continuous expectoration of purulent sputum is more typical of bronchiectasis than COPD.
- Breathlessness without productive cough or wheezing is more typical of cardiac disease or of other lung diseases such as interstitial pulmonary fibrosis.

Physical signs

The typical patient with established COPD shows some or all of the following features, but in mild disease (FEV_1 >50% of predicted) there may be no abnormal signs.

Large, barrel shaped chest (hyperinflation).

Prominent accessory respiratory muscles in neck and use of accessory muscles in respiration.

Low, flat diaphragm causing costal margin retractions on inspiration.

Diminished breath sounds, distant heart sounds.

Prolonged expiration with generalized wheezing predominantly on expiration.

Depressed liver which is not enlarged.

The 'blue bloater' type of COPD patient may also have:
- cyanosis at rest or mild exertion;
- oedema of ankles;
- crackles at lung bases; and
- loud second heart sound in pulmonary area (difficult to hear in COPD).

The 'pink puffer' type of COPD patient may also have:
- expiratory pursed-lip breathing (auto-PEEP);
- thin body build; and
- tendency to lean forward over a support to assist breathing.

N.B. Clubbing is NOT a feature of COPD and suggests either malignancy, bronchiectasis or some other type of lung disease.

Investigations

Investigations are essential to confirm the diagnosis of COPD. Any patient presenting with a history of cough, sputum production and breathlessness requires certain basic investigations (*see* Table 2.1.) which may in turn suggest the need for further investigations.

Investigation of COPD

Indication	Test
Routine (all patients)	FEV_1, FEV_1/FVC Bronchodilator response Chest radiograph TLCO/KCO
Moderate/severe COPD	Lung volumes SaO_2 and/or blood gases ECG Haemoglobin
Persistent purulent sputum	Sputum culture/sensitivity
Emphysema in young patient	α_1-Antitrypsin, genotyping if low
Assessment of bullae	CT scan
Disproportionate breathlessness	Exercise test
Suspected asthma	Trial of steroids PEF monitoring Airway responsiveness
Suspected sleep apnoea	Nocturnal sleep study

Table 2.1. COPD, chronic obstructive pulmonary disease; FEV_1, forced expiratory volume in one second; FVC, forced vital capacity; TLCO, transfer factor of carbon monoxide; KCO (TLCO/VA), transfer coefficient of carbon monoxide; SaO_2, arterial oxygen saturation; ECG, electrocardiography; CT, computed tomography.

Chest radiograph

In mild COPD the plain chest radiograph is usually normal. With advancing disease, hyperinflation (*see* Figure 2.1) manifests as large volume lungs; a low, flat diaphragm; a thin heart shadow; and an enlarged retrosternal air space on the lateral view.

Plain chest radiographs cannot diagnose mild emphysema.

When *emphysema* is prominent there is a loss of fine vascular markings, especially at the periphery of the lung, and bullae (areas of transradiency surrounded by a thin wall) may appear.

When cor pulmonale occurs, the hilar vasculature may become prominent and the heart may enlarge, especially in the antero-posterior direction.

With *infections* there may be localized infiltrates in the lungs, which should disappear with antibiotic treatment.

The following features on a plain chest radiograph are not consistent with a diagnosis of uncomplicated COPD and should raise the possibility of an alternative diagnosis:

- persistent localized infiltrate;
- persistent atelectasis;
- hilar node enlargement;
- parenchymal nodules or masses;
- pleural disease; and
- interstitial infiltrates.

Computed tomography

A computed tomography (CT) scan of the thorax is useful for demonstrating emphysema (*see* Figure 2.2) [5]. Typical appearances are areas of low attenuation

Chest radiograph of patient with COPD

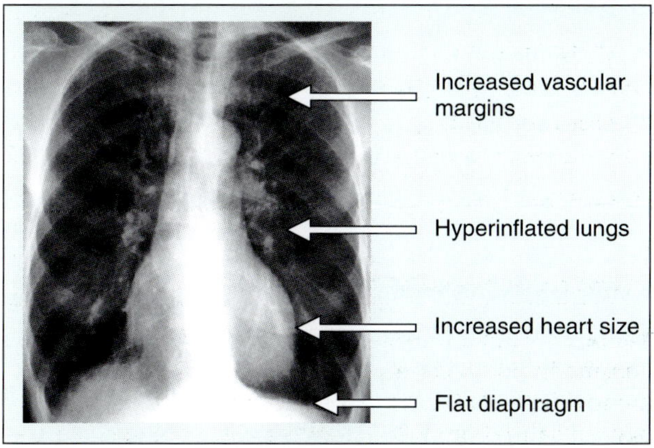

Figure 2.1. The lungs are hyperinflated, the diaphragm is flattened, vascular markings are increased and the heart size is marginally increased. COPD, chronic obstructive pulmonary disease.

Computed tomography scan of patient with emphysema

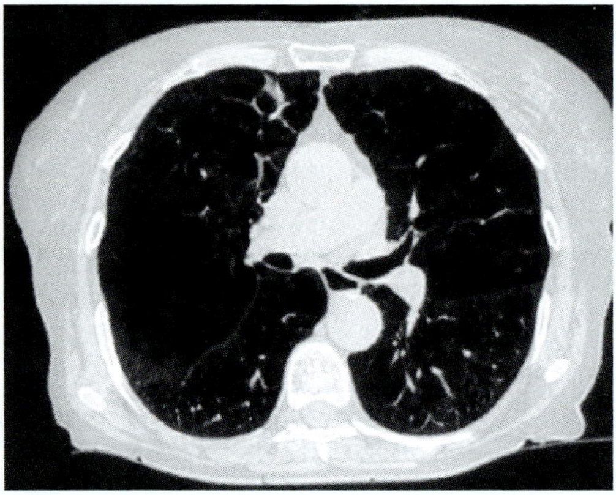

Figure 2.2. Computed tomography scan shows reduced density of the lungs with enlarged air spaces.

and bullae; attenuation and pruning of the vascular tree; and abnormal vascular configurations.

A CT scan of the lungs may be indicated as the disease progresses because:

- Most patients with COPD are heavy smokers and a small carcinoma may be difficult to diagnose on a plain chest radiograph.
- It may be impossible to distinguish between a simple infectious exacerbation of COPD and the appearance of malignancy on a plain radiograph.
- Complications of COPD such as pulmonary thromboembolism and pulmonary artery thrombosis can be detected by a CT with contrast injection, especially using spiral CT.
- CT scans can distinguish centriacinar from panacinar emphysema (although this may not yet be useful in management).
- Bronchiectasis can be diagnosed on CT scans and this may be a feature in patients with severe disease.
- CT scans are essential in order to determine the distribution of emphysema for the selection of patients for lung volume reduction surgery.

Lung function tests

Lung function tests are used for diagnosis, assessment of severity and following the course of the disease. Objective lung function tests are essential because symptoms and physical signs cannot predict disease severity. The hallmark of COPD is chronic airflow obstruction which is largely irreversible. The obstruction is particularly marked in the smaller airways due to the pathological changes of chronic obstructive bronchitis and the loss of support for their walls due to emphysema. These small airways close off during expiration, trapping gas and increasing resting lung volume (functional residual capacity [FRC]) and residual volume (RV). Emphysema may also result in an increase in total lung capacity (TLC) and loss of the alveolar surface area available for gas exchange. There are various tests that are useful in evaluating lung function in COPD (*see* Table 2.2).

Lung function test abnormalities in COPD

Lung function test	Result
FEV_1 (litres)	↓
FVC (litres)	↓
FEV_1/FVC (%)	↓
PEF (l/min)	↓
TLC (litres)	↑
FRC (litres)	↑
RV (litres)	↑
sGaw ($cmH_2O^{-1}.sec^{-1}$)	↓
TLCO (ml/min/mmHg)	↓
KCO (TLCO/VA) (ml/min/mmHg/l)	↓

Table 2.2. FEV_1, forced expiratory volume in one second; FVC, forced vital capacity; PEF, peak expiratory flow; TLC, total lung capacity; FRC, functional residual capacity; RV, residual volume; sGaw, specific airway conductance; TLCO, transfer factor of carbon monoxide; KCO (TLCO/VA), transfer coefficient of carbon monoxide.

Spirometry

The simplest and most useful measure of airways obstruction is obtained by having the patient perform a forced expiration from TLC and recording the spirogram (*see* Figure 2.3). In COPD the following changes are to be expected:

- *FEV_1* is always reduced, with progressively greater reduction as disease advances. *FEV_1 is the most useful test to assess severity and progression of COPD.* Yearly measurement of FEV_1 over at least three years is needed to define the annual rate of decline; more than 50 ml/year suggests accelerated decline.
- *Forced vital capacity* (FVC) is initially normal but is reduced as disease progresses.
- *Slow vital capacity* is more accurate than FVC because it is not limited by dynamic compression of the airways.
- *FEV_1/FVC ratio* is always less than the normal adult value of about 80% and drops further as disease progresses. It may not accurately reflect very severe COPD because FVC is then also reduced.

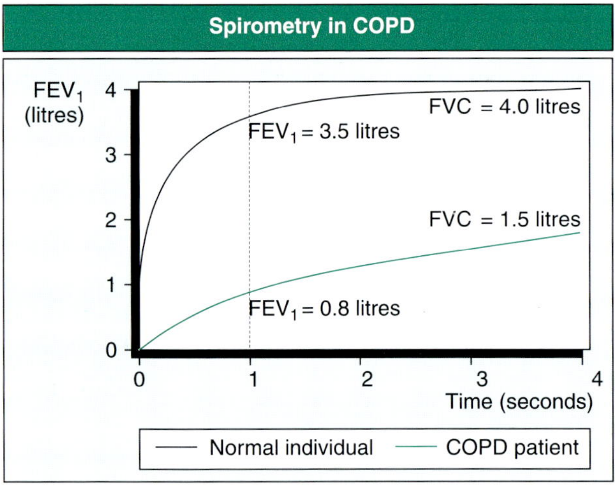

Figure 2.3. There is a marked reduction in forced expiratory volume in one second (FEV_1), forced vital capacity (FVC) and FEV_1/FVC ratio.

- *Maximum mid-expiratory flow* (MMEF) primarily reflects small airways function and is markedly reduced in patients with COPD. It has a much greater variability than FEV_1 so is less useful for routine monitoring.

Peak expiratory flow

The peak expiratory flow (PEF) test gives a crude estimate of lung function, reflecting larger airway function. PEF is very effort dependent and reduces roughly in proportion to disease severity. *It is not as useful in diagnosing COPD as it is in asthma, and it may be relatively well preserved in emphysema.* A normal PEF does not exclude COPD.

Bronchodilator response

The effect of inhaling a bronchodilator on spirometry is usually minimal with an increase less than 12% or less than 200 ml increase in FEV_1 (in patients with FEV_1 <1 litre). *A lack of bronchodilator response does not mean that bronchodilators will not have any clinical benefit in patients with COPD.*

Flow-volume loops

These provide similar information to spirometry and show a reduction in flow across the volume range, but with relatively good preservation of PEF (*see* Figure 2.4).

Lung volumes

When the disease is severe, when there is doubt about the diagnosis or when it is important to know the extent of the emphysema (eg, when considering volume reduction surgery or lung transplantation) further investigation is required. Absolute (static) lung volumes are measured by body plethysmography. Lung volumes can also be measured by inert gas dilution methods but this is unreliable because the uneven ventilation prevents good mixing of the marker gas with the gas in the lungs.

- *Total lung capacity* (TLC) may show modest increase but may be markedly increased in patients with predominant emphysema.

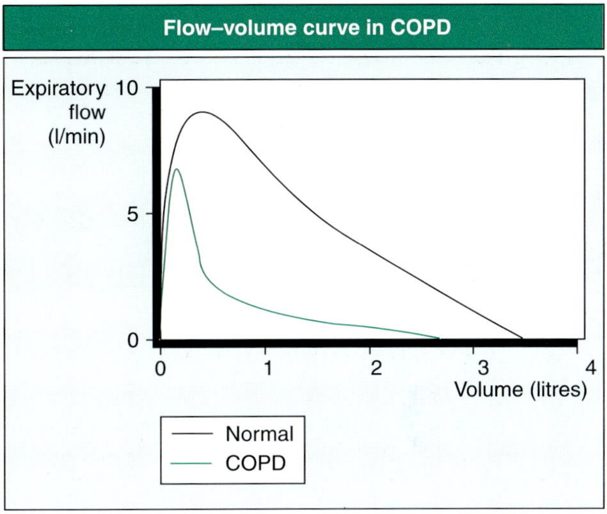

Figure 2.4. There is a marked reduction in expiratory flow with a relatively preserved peak expiratory flow. COPD, chronic obstructive pulmonary disease.

- *Residual volume* (RV) is invariably increased due to gas trapping; RV / TLC ratio is always more than 40%.
- *Functional residual capacity* (FRC) is increased as with RV but less reliable.

Airways resistance (Raw)

This measurement reflects the resistance in larger and medium sized airways. It is usually increased in COPD. Commonly expressed as its reciprocal (airway conductance [Gaw]) and related to the thoracic gas volume (Vtg) at which resistance was measured. Specific airway conductance (sGaw = Gaw / Vtg) is usually reduced.

Gas transfer (diffusing capacity)

In most patients with COPD gas transfer is relatively well preserved. When emphysema is marked, however, the surface area for gas exchange is reduced. Typically, there is a fall in the transfer factor of carbon monoxide (TLCO; and similarly of oxygen) in absolute terms and when corrected for the increased alveolar volume (transfer coefficient: KCO or TLCO / VA).

Airway responsiveness

There is an increase in responsiveness to histamine and methacholine and this is less than that seen in asthma and is related to baseline lung function. Responses to indirect stimuli such as adenosine monophosphate, sodium metabisulphite and exercise are normal, however. Bronchial challenge tests are not useful in clinical practice and should not be conducted when FEV_1 is less than 70% of the predicted normal.

Respiratory muscle function

Maximum expiratory mouth pressure is usually normal until COPD is well advanced, but maximum inspiratory pressures are reduced due to hyperinflation.

Function of skeletal muscles, such as quadriceps, may be reduced in cachectic patients.

Arterial blood gases

COPD is invariably accompanied by some degree of ventilation/perfusion (V/Q) mismatching which results in arterial hypoxia when breathing room air. In some patients there is also a degree of respiratory failure resulting in an increase in arterial partial pressures of carbon dioxide ($PaCO_2$). $PaCO_2$ increases as FEV_1 falls below 1.5 litres. In COPD patients with chronic respiratory failure there should be metabolic compensation with an elevated base excess (or bicarbonate) and relatively normal pH (7.4).

- Arterial blood gases should be measured in patients with COPD in a stable state when their condition is moderate or severe (FEV_1 <60% of that predicted).
- Pulse oximetry measures oxygen saturation (SaO_2), but is not a good guide for diagnostic purposes, since it only indicates oxygenation and does not indicate the changes in $PaCO_2$; it may be useful for following the development of hypoxia as the disease advances. If SaO_2 is less than 92%, blood gas tensions should be measured.
- Arterial blood gases should be measured during acute exacerbations of COPD to assess the degree of ventilatory failure. Because the pH is usually normal in stable COPD, the fall in pH is an indication of the severity of the exacerbation.

Exercise testing

Some patients with mild COPD may have little or no disturbance of blood gases at rest and hypoxia only appears on exercise. In others with more marked disease the decision as to whether to recommend supplemental oxygen should be made with the help of an objective evaluation of the degree of effort limitation. There are several exercise protocols in use as follows.

Progressive ergometer stress test

In this test the patient exercises on a cycle ergometer (or treadmill) with a progressively increasing work load until unable to continue further. Before undertaking an exercise test it is important to check that the patient is in a stable state, and that there is no coincident ischaemic heart disease, recent thromboembolism or cor pulmonale.

A number of parameters can be measured that reflect the nature and severity of the disturbed physiology. These include:

- maximum oxygen uptake — reduced in relation to severity of COPD;
- minute ventilation — increased in relation to severity of COPD;
- breathing reserve (maximum voluntary ventilation–maximum exercise ventilation) — reduced, patient is limited by ventilation;
- estimated dead space — increased due to V/Q mismatching;
- oxygen saturation — falls with increasing work load; and

- heart rate - normal unless there is cardiac involvement.

Oxygenation should be checked by pulse oximetry or arterial blood gases during exercise.

Six minute walk

In this test the patient is encouraged to walk as far as possible at his or her own pace for six minutes and the total distance measured is noted [6]. In a more advanced version of this test the patient is fitted with a pulse oximeter and oxygen saturation is measured throughout the test. The distance covered correlates well with lung function and diffusing capacity, but not with oxygen saturation during the walk. In a typical patient with COPD and an FEV_1 of about 1 litre or 40% of that predicted, the six-minute walk distance would be about 400 metres. There is considerable inter-subject variability which depends on emotional state, expectations and motivation. It is a valuable and simple index for following progression of the disease in the individual patient.

Shuttle test

This is similar to the walk test, but involves walking round two markers set 10 m apart and is easier to conduct in a hospital setting [7,8].

Sleep studies

Many patients with significant COPD underventilate during sleep and worsen the existing V/Q imbalance or respiratory failure [9]. This causes further hypoxia and may initiate or aggravate pulmonary hypertension and cor pulmonale. A formal sleep study with polysomnography may be indicated in those suspected of having central or obstructive sleep apnoea, but for many patients it is sufficient to perform overnight monitoring of oxygenation with pulse oximetry [10]. The greater the proportion of sleeping time spent with a saturation of less than 90%, the greater the risk of cor pulmonale. Patients without significant hypoxia when awake are unlikely to suffer as a result of desaturation during sleep, but should this cause problems, supplemental oxygen therapy during sleep may be needed.

Blood tests

Blood tests, other than of arterial blood gas measurements, are of limited importance in the investigation and management of COPD, although they may be indicated from time to time.

- *Polycythaemia* (haematocrit >47% in females or >52% in males) is an indication of chronic hypoxia and is most common in the 'blue bloater' type of COPD.
- Electrolyte imbalance may occur in patients with cor pulmonale, especially in those treated with diuretics in whom *hypokalaemia* may be a problem.
- Estimation of α_1-AT levels is indicated in the initial evaluation of a patient with COPD, especially if the patient is younger than 45 years and emphysema is prominent.
- Estimation of the α_1-AT phenotype by Pi genotyping is indicated if the α_1-AT levels are very low or if a variant of the disorder is suspected.

Trial of steroids

COPD by definition is a form of obstructive lung disease with a poor degree of reversibility and in these patients the functional response to an inhaled bronchodilator is usually less than 15% (*see* Figure 2.5) [11]. However, there are also some patients with chronic asthma whose response to bronchodilator inhalation is poor, and it is important to distinguish the conditions since their management is quite different. For this reason, it is worth performing a trial of corticosteroid therapy in all patients with significant obstructive lung disease, unless a definite diagnosis has already been established. Approximately 10% of patients with COPD respond to corticosteroids [12]; these patients probably have concomitant asthma and should be continued on inhaled steroids. The stages in performing a steroid trial are as follows:

1. estimate airways obstruction (spirometry) before and after bronchodilator;
2. perform a six-minute walk or similar exercise test;
3. ideally, measure morning PEF daily for two weeks to obtain baseline values;

Effect of oral prednisolone on lung function in COPD or asthma

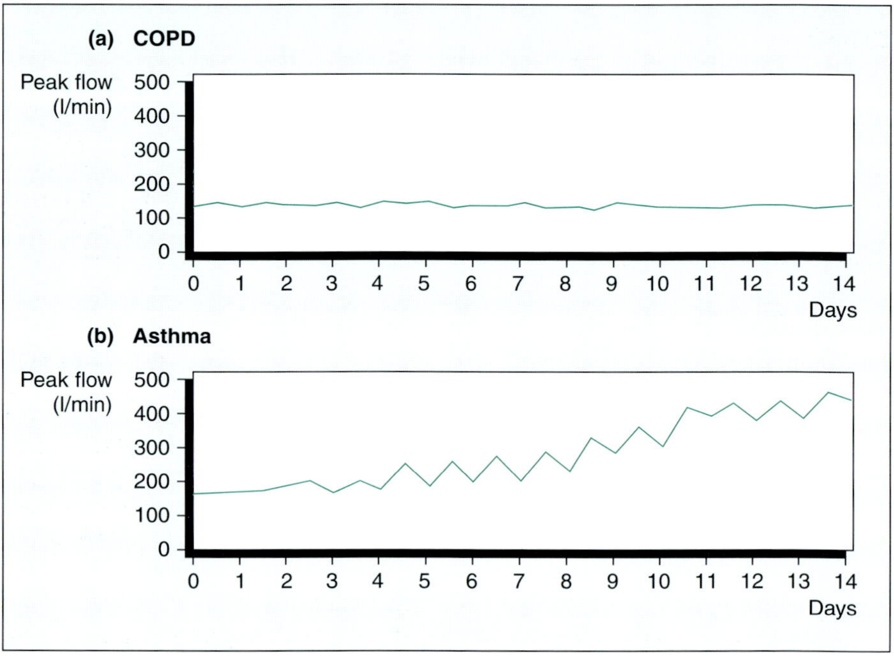

Figure 2.5. Oral prednisolone (30 mg daily for 14 days) has no effect on lung function in a patient with chronic obstructive pulmonary disease (COPD) (a), but produces a marked improvement in a patient with asthma (b). Adapted from [11].

4. give prednisolone 30–40 mg daily for two weeks and measure morning PEF daily; and
5. repeat all lung function and exercise measurements.

Improvement in all parameters to within normal range suggests that the diagnosis is asthma, not COPD. Modest improvement, but not to normal levels may be an indication that corticosteroid therapy could help the patient with COPD; these patients have a better prognosis [13]. No improvement suggests that corticosteroids have no place in management and may produce unwanted side effects. Beware the euphoric effect of corticosteroids, which may make the patient feel better in the absence of any objective improvement.

Sputum examination

Routine culture of sputum is of no value. Sputum cytology shows a neutrophilia even in patients with stable disease, but this is of no clinical use [14].

Electrocardiography

ECG is useful for detecting coexisting ischaemic heart disease. It is insensitive to detection of right ventricular hypertrophy and criteria for detection of hypertrophy are attenuated by hyperinflation.

Exhaled gases

Monitoring of exhaled gases is a new non-invasive way to monitor pulmonary inflammation, and is now a research tool, but may be introduced as a clinical measurement in the future [15]. Exhaled nitric oxide (NO) has been studied in greatest detail. In normal cigarette smokers and most patients with COPD exhaled NO levels are lower than normal [16], whereas in asthma levels are high in patients not treated with inhaled corticosteroids. An elevated level of NO in patients with COPD therefore indicates coexistent asthma and predicts a response to corticosteroid therapy [17].

Quality of life

COPD may have a major impact on the quality of life. Validated questionnaires, such as the St George's Respiratory Questionnaire which is specifically designed for patients with COPD, quantify symptoms and the impact of the disease on daily living [18,19]. Quality of life questionnaires assess the overall impact of COPD on daily living and may be more sensitive than physiological measurements in assessing the severity of disease and its response to treatment, although they are time consuming to perform. These are, however, very useful in clinical trials of COPD therapies.

Dyspnoea scores

Simple breathlessness (dyspnoea) scores may be useful as they help predict patients suitable for pulmonary rehabilitation and lung volume reduction surgery [20]. The most widely used score is the Medical Research Council (MRC) Modified Dyspnoea Score (*see* Table 2.3).

MRC Modified Dyspnoea Scale	
Grade	**Findings**
0	No breathlessness
1	Breathlessness with strenuous exercise
2	Short of breath when hurrying on a level or walking up a slight hill
3	Walks slower than people of same age on the level or stops for breath while walking at own pace on the level
4	Stops for breath after walking 100 yards
5	Too breathless to leave the house or breathless when dressing or undressing

Table 2.3. MRC, Medical Research Council.

Special types of COPD

In some patients COPD is unrelated or only partly related to cigarette smoking and COPD may also occur in young people due to a variety of causes.

α_1-Antitrypsin deficiency

This is due to a severe reduction in hepatic production of the major antiprotease in lung parenchyma as a result of a genetic defect [21,22]. This renders the lung susceptible to the destructive effects of neutrophil elastase and other endogenous proteases and results in severe panacinar emphysema, especially in smokers. This type of COPD appears at a much younger age (in the 3rd to 4th decade) and may even appear in childhood. The condition is rare, accounting for less than 1% of patients with COPD, and only occurs in homozygous carriers of the defective genes. Heterozygotes are usually healthy.

Primary ciliary dyskinesia

This is due to a defect in the ultrastructure of cilia throughout the body, which commonly results in chronic sinusitis, chronic otitis and COPD [23]. Males are sterile due to immotile spermatozoa. In one form of the disease there may be dextrocardia and bronchiectasis (Kartagener's syndrome) but most patients have a mild type of COPD.

Differential diagnosis

The differential diagnosis of COPD compared with other types of chronic obstructive lung disease is based on the clinical and functional parameters discussed in this chapter. Differentiation from the genetic disorders considered above is usually straightforward and the problem lies in the differentiation between COPD, asthma, heart failure and bronchiectasis in the older patient. In all these conditions, cough and breathlessness are common, while sputum production is prominent in COPD and bronchiectasis. These conditions are usually easy to differentiate.

Congestive heart failure

- Fine basal crackles.
- Characteristic chest radiograph with dilated heart, upper lobe blood diversion, pulmonary oedema.
- Spirometry shows no obstructive pattern.

Bronchiectasis

- Copious purulent sputum.
- Coarse crackles, may be localized.
- Confirmed by CT scan.

Obliterative bronchiolitis

- Younger patients, non-smokers.
- May have rheumatoid arthritis/fume exposure/lung transplantation.
- CT scan on expiration shows hypodense (black) areas.

Chronic asthma

- Variable symptoms.
- Early onset.
- Non-smoker.
- Response to bronchodilators and/or corticosteroids.

Tuberculosis

- Onset at all ages.
- Chest radiographs show lung infiltrate or nodular lesions and fibrosis.
- High local prevalence (developing countries).

Diffuse panbronchiolitis [24]

- Mainly in Japan.
- Most patients are male and non-smokers.
- Chronic sinusitis commonly associated.
- Characteristic chest radiograph and CT scan with diffuse small centrilobular nodular opacities and hyperinflation.
- Responds to treatment with macrolide antibiotics, such as erythromycin.

Disease progression

Since COPD typically results from irreversible damage to the alveoli and smaller airways due to smoking, there is no chance of completely curing the disease, which usually follows a slow but progressive downhill course over many years. If the patient stops smoking, the rate of decline of lung function is substantially slowed.

The typical course of COPD is characterized by:

- breathlessness that initially occurs on exercise, but later at rest; is progressive (worsens over time) and persistent (present every day); is worse during respiratory infections;
- cough and sputum initially in the morning but later all day (seldom only nocturnal);
- acute respiratory infections with increasing frequency, especially in winter;
- hypoxia initially on exercise, later during sleep and even at rest by day;
- chronic respiratory failure and cor pulmonale; and
- terminal acute respiratory failure.

Classification of disease severity

COPD is arbitrarily classified into levels of severity (*see* Table 2.4), although these arbitrary differences vary between guidelines.

Classification of COPD by disease severity (GOLD guidelines)

Disease severity	Lung function	Symptoms
Stage 0: at risk	FEV_1 >80%	Normal spirometry Chronic symptoms (cough and sputum production).
Stage I: mild	FEV_1/FVC <70% FEV_1 ≤80%	Usually chronic cough and sputum Little or no breathlessness
Stage II: moderate	FEV_1/FVC <70% 30% ≤FEV_1<80%	Progression of symptoms with SOB on exertion. Exacerbations (usually when FEV_1 <50%)
Stage III: severe	FEV_1/FVC <70% FEV_1 <30%	Severe symptoms Respiratory failure Clinical symptoms of right heart failure

Table 2.4. COPD, chronic obstructive pulmonary disease. FEV_1, forced expiratory volume in one second; FVC, forced vital capacity. GOLD, Global Initiative for Chronic Obstructive Lung Disease; SOB, shortness of breath.

References

1. O'Donnell DM, Moynihan J, Finlay GA *et al.* **Exhaled nitric oxide and bronchoalveolar lavage nitrite/nitrate in active pulmonary sarcoidosis.** *Am J Respir Crit Care Med* 1997; **156**:1892–1896.

2. Schols AM, Slangen J, Volovics L *et al.* **Weight loss is a reversible factor in the prognosis of chronic obstructive pulmonary disease.** *Am J Respir Crit Care Med* 1998; **157**:1791–1797.

3. Wouters EF. **Nutrition and metabolism in COPD.** *Chest* 2000; **117**(Suppl):274S–80S.

4. van Ede L, Yzermans CJ, Brouwer HJ. **Prevalence of depression in patients with chronic obstructive pulmonary disease: a systematic review.** *Thorax* 1999; **54**:688–692.

5. O'Brien C, Guest PJ, Hill SL *et al.* **Physiological and radiological characterisation of patients diagnosed with chronic obstructive pulmonary disease in primary care.** *Thorax* 2000; **55**:635–642.

6. Enright PL, Sherrill DL. **Reference equations for the six-minute walk in healthy adults.** *Am J Respir Crit Care Med* 1998; **158**:1384–1387.

7. Singh SJ, Morgan MD, Hardman AE *et al.* **Comparison of oxygen uptake during a conventional treadmill test and the shuttle walking test in chronic airflow limitation.** *Eur Respir J* 1994; **7**:2016–2020.

8. Revill SM, Morgan MD, Singh SJ *et al.* **The endurance shuttle walk: a new field test for the assessment of endurance capacity in chronic obstructive pulmonary disease.** *Thorax* 1999; **54**:213–222.

9. Brown LK. **Sleep-related disorders and chronic obstructive pulmonary disease.** *Respir Care Clin N Am* 1998; **4**:493–512.

10. Weitzenblum E, Chaouat A, Charpentier C *et al.* **Sleep-related hypoxaemia in chronic obstructive pulmonary disease: causes, consequences and treatment.** *Respiration* 1997; **64**:187–193.

11. Weir DC, Burge PS. **Assessment of reversibility of airway obstruction in patients with chronic obstructive airways disease.** *Thorax* 1990; **45**:907–908.

12. Callahan CM, Dittus RS, Katz BP. **Oral corticosteroid therapy for patients with stable chronic obstructive pulmonary disease. A meta-analysis.** *Ann Intern Med* 1991; **114**:216–223.

13. Davies L, Nisar M, Pearson MG *et al.* **Oral corticosteroid trials in the management of stable chronic obstructive pulmonary disease.** *QJM* 1999; **92**:395–400.

14. Keatings VM, Collins PD, Scott DM *et al.* **Differences in interleukin-8 and tumor necrosis factor-alpha in induced sputum from patients with chronic obstructive pulmonary disease or asthma.** *Am J Respir Crit Care Med* 1996; **153**:530–534.

15. Kharitonov SA, Barnes PJ. **Exhaled markers of pulmonary disease.** *Am J Respir Crit Care Med* 2001; **163**:1693–1772.

16. Maziak W, Loukides S, Culpitt S *et al.* **Exhaled nitric oxide in chronic obstructive pulmonary disease.** *Am J Respir Crit Care Med* 1998; **157**:998–1002.

17. Papi A, Romagnoli M, Baraldo S *et al.* **Partial reversibility of airflow limitation and increased exhaled NO and sputum eosinophilia in chronic obstructive pulmonary disease.** *Am J Respir Crit Care Med* 2000; **162**:1773–1777.

18. Jones PW. **Quality of life, symptoms and pulmonary function in asthma: long-term treatment with nedocromil sodium examined in a controlled multicentre trial.** *Eur Respir J* 1994; **7**:55–62.

19. Spencer S, Calverley PM, Sherwood BP *et al.* **Health status deterioration in patients with chronic obstructive pulmonary disease.** *Am J Respir Crit Care Med* 2001; **163**:122–128.

20. Bestall JC, Paul EA, Garrod R *et al.* **Usefulness of the Medical Research Council (MRC) dyspnoea scale as a measure of disability in patients with chronic obstructive pulmonary disease.** *Thorax* 1999; **54**:581–586.

21. Crystal RG, Brantly ML, Hubbard RC *et al.* **The alpha 1-antitrypsin gene and its mutations. Clinical consequences and strategies for therapy.** *Chest* 1989; **95**:196–208.

22. Mahadeva R, Lomas DA. **Genetics and respiratory disease. 2. Alpha 1-antitrypsin deficiency, cirrhosis and emphysema.** *Thorax* 1998; **53**:501–505.

23. Bush A, Cole P, Hariri M *et al.* **Primary ciliary dyskinesia: diagnosis and standards of care.** *Eur Respir J* 1998; **12**:982–988.

24. Sugiyama Y. **Diffuse panbronchiolitis.** *Clin Chest Med* 1993; **14**:765–772.

Chapter 3

Drugs used in the management of COPD

Bronchodilators

Bronchodilators (or relievers) give relatively rapid relief of symptoms and are believed to work predominantly by relaxation of airway smooth muscle (although several other effects on the airways may contribute to their therapeutic effects). They are currently the mainstay of management of COPD. Bronchodilators are traditionally assessed by demonstrating a short-term increase in FEV_1 or PEF, but in COPD these changes are very small (<10%), yet patients may feel symptomatic benefit [1]. This may be because bronchodilators lead to deflation of the lung, with a reduction in residual volume. This makes breathing more comfortable and dyspnoea is lessened [2]. The deflation may also lead to improvement in exercise performance [3]. Bronchodilator efficacy in COPD may therefore best be judged by improvement in symptoms, rather than through the traditional lung function tests used to assess bronchodilator efficacy in asthma.

Anticholinergics

Anticholinergics are the bronchodilators of choice for COPD and in many studies they have been shown to be more effective than β_2-agonists [4,5]. The most commonly used drugs are ipratropium bromide and oxitropium bromide. A new once daily anticholinergic tiotropium bromide is now approved for use in COPD in several countries (*see* 'Tiotropium bromide' section later).

Mode of action

Anticholinergics act as muscarinic receptor antagonists, inhibit cholinergic reflex bronchoconstriction and reduce vagal cholinergic tone, which is the main reversible component in COPD (*see* Figures 3.1 and 3.2). Normal airways have a small degree of vagal cholinergic tone, but because the airways are patent this has no perceptible effect and does not reduce airflow. When the airways are irreversibly narrowed in COPD vagal cholinergic tone has a much greater effect on airway resistance for geometric reasons, so when this increased constriction is relieved by an anticholinergic drug there is a perceptible improvement in airflow. In addition, anticholinergics may reduce mucus hypersecretion [6]. Anticholinergics have no effect on pulmonary vessels, and therefore no fall in PaO_2, as may sometimes be seen with β_2-agonists and theophylline.

Recommended use

Regular treatment either as metered dose inhaler (MDI), dry powder inhaler (DPI) or nebulizer three or four times is recommended. Combination inhalers with an anticholinergic and a short-acting β_2-agonist (such as Combivent: ipratropium bromide and salbutamol) are very useful, giving a greater speed of onset of action and additive bronchodilator effects [7].

Side effects

Side effects are very uncommon because anticholinergics act topically and there is virtually no systemic absorption.

Cholinergic nerves in the airway

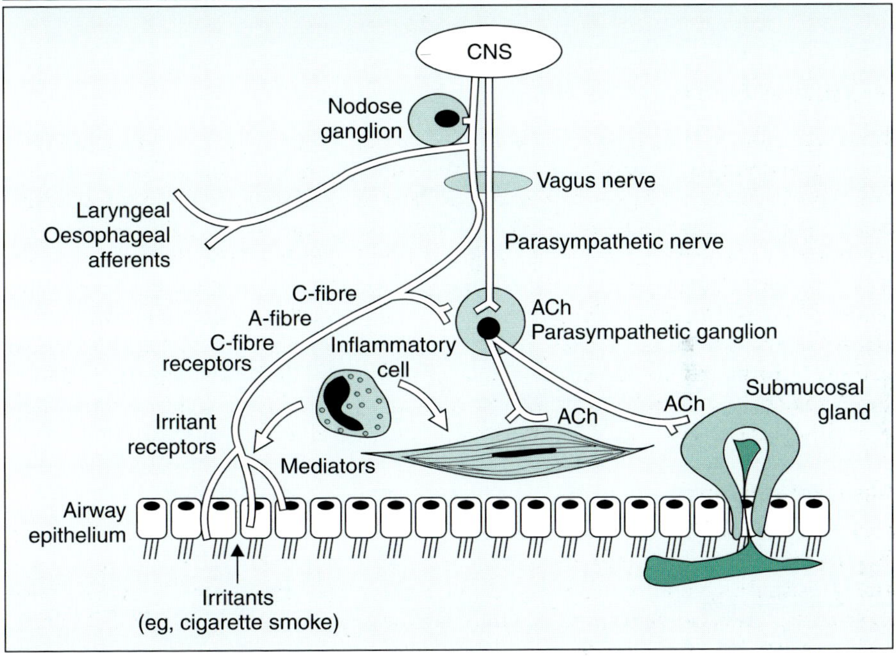

Figure 3.1. Cholinergic fibres in the vagus nerve relay in parasympathetic ganglia in the airway wall and short post-ganglionic pathways release acetylcholine (ACh) to cause bronchoconstriction and mucus secretion. Cholinergic pathways may be activated by inflammatory mediators and cigarette smoke. CNS, central nervous system.

- Paradoxical bronchoconstriction (usually due to additives in nebulizer solution).
- Glaucoma (especially with nebulized drug when used without mouthpiece in elderly patients).
- Bitter taste.
- Systemic effects such as dry mouth, urinary retention, constipation: very rare.

Short-acting inhaled β_2-agonists

Mode of action

β_2-Agonists have several beneficial effects on the airways in COPD (*see* Figure 3.3). These drugs acts on airway smooth muscle causing a relaxation in large and small airways. They act as functional antagonists and reverse bronchoconstriction irrespective of cause. Experimentally, they reduce plasma exudation and cholinergic reflexes. They also increase mucociliary clearance (when it is reduced), but have no effect on chronic inflammation. Recent evidence suggests that β-agonists may reduce

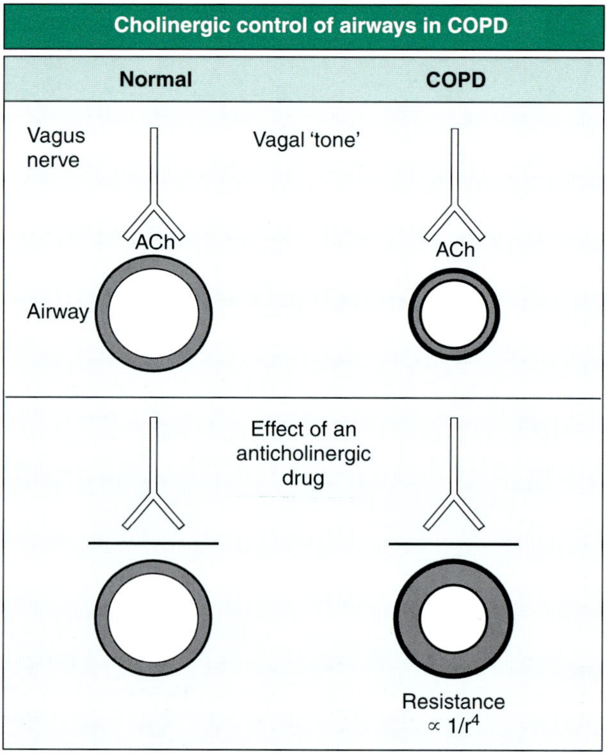

Figure 3.2. Normally there is a certain amount of cholinergic tone. This is exaggerated in chronic obstructive pulmonary disease (COPD) because of geometric factors related to the fixed narrowing of the airways, so that airway resistance improves to a greater extent than in normal airway with an anticholinergic drug.

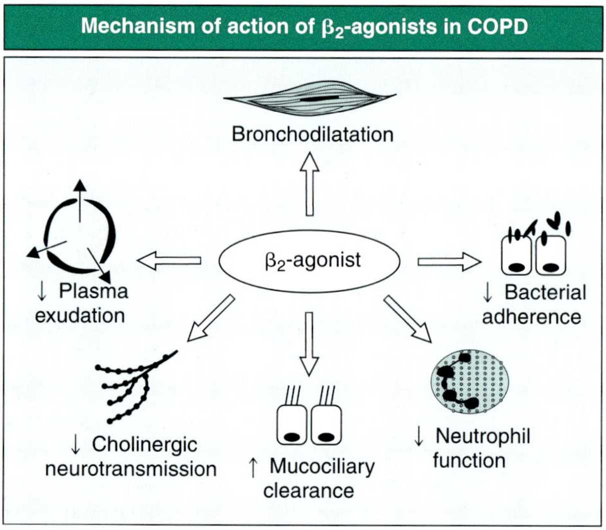

Figure 3.3. Although their primary action is likely to be on airway smooth muscle, there are several additional effects of β_2-agonists that may be beneficial.

adherence of bacteria to airway epithelial cells and this may reduce infective exacerbations [8]. There is some evidence that β_2-agonists may increase the ventilatory drive to hypercapnia (but not to hypoxia) [9].

Recommended use in COPD

β_2-Agonists are recommended for immediate relief of symptoms. Ideally should not be used regularly (as tolerance to their protective effects occurs), although in patients with severe COPD regular nebulized β_2-agonists may be indicated.

Side effects

- Muscle tremor (direct effect on skeletal muscle β_2-receptors) — more common in elderly patients.
- Tachycardia (direct effect on atrial β_2-receptors, reflex effect from increased peripheral vasodilatation via β_2-receptors).
- Hypokalaemia (direct effect on skeletal muscle uptake of potassium via β_2-receptors) — usually a small effect and of no clinical significance.
- Restlessness.
- Hypoxaemia (increased V/Q mismatch due to pulmonary vasodilatation).

Long-acting inhaled β_2-agonists

Salmeterol and formoterol give bronchodilatation and protection against bronchoconstriction for more than 12 hours. There is increasing evidence that these drugs are useful as additional bronchodilators in patients with COPD [10]. These drugs may improve symptoms, quality of life and exercise performance [11]. They have a similar efficacy to anticholinergics and should be considered as supplementary [12]. For regular therapy long-acting inhaled β_2-agonists should be administered twice daily. Side effects are usually only a problem if high doses are used. If the inhibitory effect of β_2-agonists on bacterial adhesion is relevant *in vivo* they may also reduce the frequency of infective exacerbations [8].

Oral β_2-agonists

Although inhaled β_2-agonists are preferred, some elderly patients have problems with inhalers. Slow-release oral β_2-agonist preparations, such as bambuterol and slow-release salbutamol, are available. The advantage of these preparations is that they may treat peripheral airways more effectively, but the disadvantage is that side effects are much more frequent that with inhaled preparations. Bambuterol is a prodrug that is slowly metabolized to terbutaline and is effective as a once daily preparation in COPD [13]. In asthma it appears to be as effective as inhaled salmeterol used twice daily [14,15].

Theophylline

Theophylline is a useful additional bronchodilator in patients with COPD, and oral administration has the advantage of treating small airways [16]. It may have additional properties such as effects on mucociliary clearance and on respiratory muscles that are useful (*see* Figure 3.4). It may also have anti-inflammatory effects in COPD with an inhibitory effect on neutrophilic inflammation [17]. The major limitation to the use of theophylline is its side effects.

Mode of action

Theophylline acts through phosphodiesterase inhibition (increasing cyclic AMP and cyclic GMP levels). This effect is important for bronchodilator action and may also be important in reducing neutrophilic inflammation [17]. The drug also has some adenosine receptor antagonism, which accounts for some of the side effects, but there is little evidence that this is relevant for bronchodilator effects. Theophylline increases adrenaline secretion, but this is unlikely to account for the effects in COPD. A further action is prostaglandin inhibition, which is probably unimportant in COPD. Theophylline inhibits calcium entry and release and phosphoinositide hydrolysis. It is difficult to explain all of the beneficial effects of theophylline through these mechanisms alone, as many only occur at concentrations higher than those used therapeutically. Theophylline, therefore, may have additional unknown modes of action.

Recommended use in COPD

Theophylline is recommended as an additional bronchodilator in patients not controlled on regular inhaled anticholinergics. It is useful in patients who have respiratory problems at night. A slow-release preparation should be given twice daily, with a higher evening dose to give steady state plasma concentrations of 10–20 mg/l. Theophylline may give good symptomatic improvement without any change in spirometry; this may be due to lung deflation and a reduction in residual volume

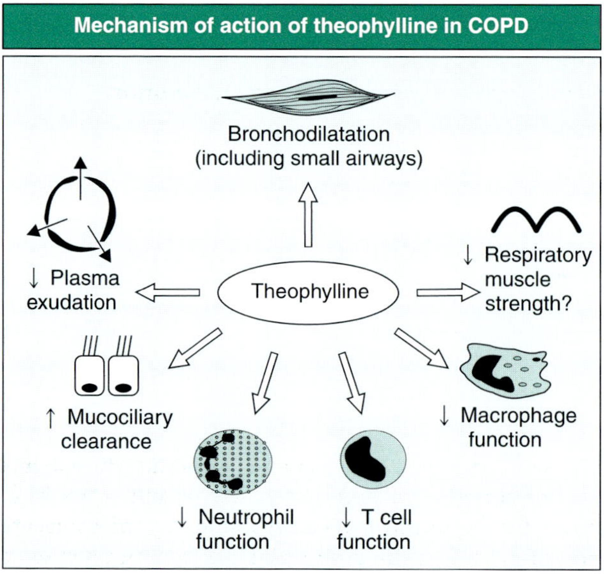

Figure 3.4. There may be several mechanisms of action of this drug. COPD, chronic obstructive pulmonary disease.

[16]. While not as effective a bronchodilator as salmeterol, theophylline has an additive effect when the two drugs are used together [18].

Side effects

Side effects are related to plasma concentration, although some patients may be particularly susceptible to side effects. They may be reduced by slowly increasing the dose when the drug is introduced. Side effects include:

- nausea and vomiting;
- headache;
- restlessness;
- gastro-oesophageal reflux;
- diuresis;
- cardiac arrhythmias (usually plasma concentration >20 mg/l); and
- epileptic seizures (usually plasma concentration >30 mg/l).

Clearance of theophylline

Therapeutic effect is related to plasma concentration, which affected by several factors that alter clearance. If in doubt, measure plasma concentration.

Increased clearance (increase dose)

- Enzyme induction (rifampicin, phenobarbitone, ethanol).
- Smoking (tobacco, marijuana).
- Childhood.
- High protein, low carbohydrate diet.
- Barbecued meat.

Decreased clearance (decrease dose)

- Enzyme inhibition (cimetidine, erythromycin, ciprofloxacin, allopurinol, ketoconazole).
- Congestive heart failure.
- Liver disease.
- Pneumonia.
- Viral infection and vaccination.
- High carbohydrate diet.

Antibiotics

Since infection is often the cause of progression or acute deterioration in patients with COPD, the combating of infection by the appropriate use of antibiotics is an important part of therapy. In fact, the organisms that cause pulmonary infections are often the same as those found normally in the upper respiratory tract and it may be difficult to know if a pathogen isolated from the sputum is responsible for the exacerbation. For most of the time the sputum in COPD is mucoid, but becomes yellow or green with exacerbations of infection, and when this occurs it is usual to begin empirical antibiotic therapy. Purulence of sputum is due to an increase in degranulating neutrophils and may not necessarily imply bacterial infection. Indeed, many exacerbations of COPD are likely to be due to upper respiratory tract virus infections, such as rhinovirus, corona virus and parainfluenza virus [19]. This means that antibiotics are often used inappropriately, but it is difficult to tell clinically whether an infection is viral or bacterial in origin. In a meta-analysis of placebo-controlled trials of antibiotics for COPD, there was a small but significant difference in PEF between patients treated with antibiotics and placebo [20].

The common bacterial organisms responsible for exacerbations of COPD include *Streptococcus pneumoniae, Haemophilus influenzae, Moraxella catarrhalis, Mycoplasma pneumoniae* (less common).

The choice of antibiotic depends upon the likely organisms, the likely sensitivity of the organisms in the community, the tolerance of the patient for the drug, and the response to treatment (*see* Table 3.1.)

The treatment of choice in the community has often been either amoxycillin or co-trimoxamole (Septrin). Co-trimoxamole is not recommended as development of resistance is common and side effects due to the sulphonamide component are relatively common. Further, because many strains of *H. influenzae* are now β-lactamase producers and hence resistant to ampicillin/amoxycillin, the treatment for initial therapy commonly lies between amoxycillin with clavulanic acid (Augmentin); erythromycin or other macrolides (clarithromycin, azithromycin); a cephalosporin (eg, cefaclor); or a tetracycline (eg, doxycycline).

There are advantages and disadvantages to each drug and the choice may finally be based on finding out which drug works for a given patient. Cost is also a factor and

Sensitivity of the common organisms found in COPD to antibiotics

Antibiotic	*S. pneumoniae*	*H. influenzae*	*M. catarrhalis*
Amoxycillin	S	S/R	R
Amoxycillin/clavulanic acid	S	S	S
Erythromycin	S	P	S
Cefaclor	P	P	P
Doxycycline	P	P	S
Co-trimoxazole	P	S	S
Clarithromycin	S	P	S
Azithromycin	S	P	S

Table 3.1. COPD, chronic obstructive pulmonary disease; S, fully sensitive; P, partially sensitive; R, resistant.

there is no justification for using an expensive drug when a cheaper one works just as well. In most cases, the choice usually falls between amoxycillin, amoxycillin with clavulanic acid or doxycycline for the typical ambulatory patient.

The antibiotic should be given in full therapeutic doses for a course lasting about 10–14 days except for clarithromycin and azithromycin which are given for three days. Treatment is then stopped provided the patient has responded. If there has been a poor response, a change of antibiotic may be indicated, usually to one of the newer broad-spectrum agents such as clarithromycin if this has not already been tried. Continuous antibiotic administration is not recommended in COPD as this has not been shown to alter the course of the disease and is likely to lead to an increase in resistant organisms.

Oxygen therapy

Poor oxygenation is one of the fundamental problems of COPD, and supplementary oxygen is an important part of therapy in patients with severe disease [21]. Controlled oxygen is used in the treatment of acute exacerbations in all patients who are hospitalized. Long-term oxygen therapy (LTOT, domiciliary oxygen) is indicated in selected patients with COPD [22,23]. Two large multicentre trials have demonstrated that long-term oxygen administration (>15 h daily) prolong survival (by approximately 30%) in patients with COPD [24,25]. The goal of oxygen therapy is to increase PaO_2 to above 60 mmHg or an oxygen saturation of over 90%; increasing PaO_2 above 60 mmHg has little further benefit and increases risk for carbon dioxide retention [26].

It should be noted that LTOT does not improve survival in patients with mild-to-moderate hypoxaemia [27].

Short-term oxygen therapy

Oxygen is delivered during an acute exacerbation via a Venturi mask, which gives precise control of the inspired oxygen concentration (24% for initial therapy). Nasal prongs (flow at 1 l/min) may also be used as these are more comfortable, but it is more difficult to precisely control inspired oxygen concentration. The major mechanism of hypoxaemia in acute exacerbations is ventilation–perfusion inequality and this is correctable with a relatively small increase in inspired oxygen. Indeed, failure to increase PaO_2 by more than 60 mmHg with 24% oxygen implies some other reason for hypoxaemia, such as pneumonia, pulmonary embolism or pneumothorax. Arterial blood gases or saturation should be checked before and 30 minutes after initiation of controlled oxygen therapy. Oxygen concentration should be adjusted to give a PaO_2 of 60 mmHg or saturation of over 90% without an increase in $PaCO_2$ or reduction in pH.

Effect of long-term oxygen therapy

- Improvement in exercise capacity (increased endurance).
- Reduction in dyspnoea.

- Reduction in pulmonary hypertension, by reducing hypoxic pulmonary vasoconstriction.
- Reduction in haematocrit by reducing erythropoietin levels.
- Improved quality of life and neuropsychiatric function.
- Reduction in severe desaturation episodes during sleep.

There are three methods of providing domiciliary oxygen therapy: long-term, low-dose oxygen (LTOT) for patients with chronic respiratory failure; portable oxygen therapy for exercise-related hypoxia and dyspnoea; and short-burst oxygen therapy for temporary relief of symptoms.

Selection of patients for LTOT

In the UK, guidelines have been drawn up by the Department of Health for the provision of LTOT [28]. *LTOT should never be considered in patients who continue to smoke.* All patients should be assessed by a pulmonary specialist.

Absolute indications are stable COPD with hypoxaemia and oedema; FEV_1 less than 1.5 litres, FVC less than 2.0 litres; and PaO_2 less than 55 mmHg (<7.3 kPa), $PaCO_2$ more than 45 mmHg (>6 kPa); *and* stability demonstrated over three weeks on optimal therapy.

Relative indications are absolute indications but without oedema or $PaCO_2$ more than 45 mmHg, and palliative treatment (symptom relief).

Portable oxygen is indicated in patients who desaturate during exercise and its efficacy needs to be assessed during a treadmill or six-minute walk test with the patient wearing a portable oxygen cylinder. Portable oxygen may also be indicated in patients with severe exercise limitation irrespective of oxygen desaturation. *Portable oxygen may also be needed in such patients during commercial airline flights (provided by airline).*

Oxygen supply

There are several ways of providing supplementary oxygen:

- *Compressed gas cylinders* containing 100% oxygen are inconvenient because regular delivery is needed and the cylinders are large and heavy, but are still the most widely used method in the UK. The cylinders are fitted with flow meters that are either medium (2 l/min) or high (4 l/min).
- *Oxygen concentrators* are the most economic and convenient way of delivering LTOT at home [29].
- *Liquid oxygen* is the most portable but most expensive form of supplementary oxygen. A lightweight device weighing 3 kg can deliver oxygen for 14 hours at 2 l/min. Liquid oxygen is not available on prescription in the UK.

Oxygen may be delivered by several devices:

- *Face masks*: tight fitting masks are the most efficient devices, but are uncomfortable and inconvenient for long-term use.

- *Nasal cannulae* are the most commonly used means of oxygen delivery and usually have no problems. A flow of 1.5–2.5 l/min is usually adequate to achieve a PaO_2 more than 60 mmHg (>8 kPa).
- *Trans-tracheal oxygen therapy* (TTOT), by means of a trans-tracheal catheter, may be useful in some patients who cannot tolerate face masks or nasal cannulae, but catheters have to be removed and cleaned frequently.
- *Pulsed delivery systems* use a thermistor or pressure valve to deliver oxygen only during the beginning of inspiration. These devices are expensive but reduce the amount of oxygen used by over one-third.

Other drug therapies

Although bronchodilator therapy is the mainstay of treatment in COPD, other treatments are commonly used.

Corticosteroids

COPD is defined by a lack of response to oral steroids in a short-term trial. In many patients a formal trial of steroids is important to exclude chronic asthma. The role of inhaled steroids in COPD patients is currently unknown. Anecdotally, some patients seem to do well, and in some studies improvement in exercise tolerance has been demonstrated. Some patients with COPD have coexisting asthma and show a response; these patients should be labelled as asthmatics and treated with long-term-inhaled corticosteroids. However, little or no convincing effect of long-term inhaled steroids on lung function has been found [30].

Cellular effects of corticosteroids

Theoretically, it might be expected that inhaled steroids would be beneficial in the long term if they suppress the inflammatory response in the airways by reduction of neutrophilic inflammation; inhibition of cytokine synthesis — including TNF-α and IL-8 [31]; inhibition of macrophage activation; increased synthesis of SLPI [32]; and decreased secretion of mucus.

However, these effects have not been demonstrated in COPD with either oral or inhaled corticosteroids, with no changes in neutrophil counts, neutrophil activation markers, inflammatory cytokines or proteases [33,34] (*see* Figure 3.5). Indeed, there may be a resistance to the anti-inflammatory effects of corticosteroids in COPD, because corticosteroids inhibit the expression of cytokines in normal persons and patients with asthma that are not inhibited in patients with COPD. Cigarette smoke and oxidative stress appear to interfere with the molecular mechanism of action of corticosteroids [35].

Long-term trials of inhaled corticosteroids in COPD

Four long-term studies have examined the use of long-term inhaled corticosteroids on the progression of COPD.

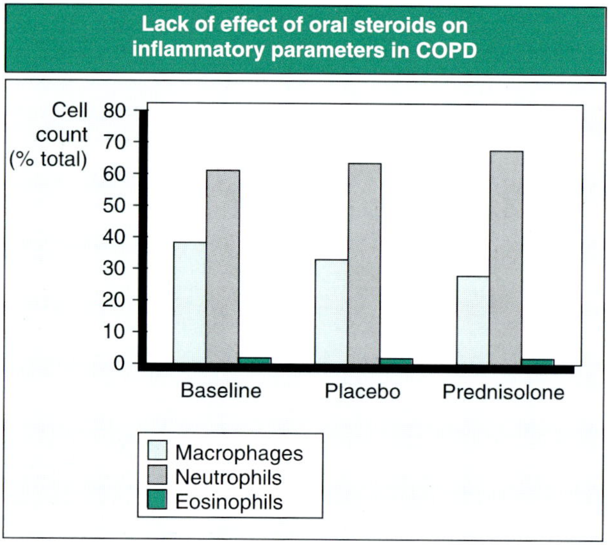

Figure 3.5. Oral prednisolone (30 mg for 14 days) was found to have no effect on inflammatory cells in induced sputum of patients with chronic obstructive pulmonary disease (COPD). Adapted from [34].

- The Copenhagen Lung Study investigated a similar group of patients with mild asthma from a single population and found no benefit of inhaled budesonide (800 μg daily) compared with placebo over three years [36].
- The EUROSCOP study investigated patients with mild COPD and compared budesonide 800 μg daily with placebo over three years of therapy. There was no significant change in the rate of decline in FEV_1 [37].
- The ISOLDE study investigated a group of patients with more severe illness and demonstrated no effect of fluticasone propionate (1000 μg daily) on the rate of decline in lung function over three years, although there was some improvement in the quality of life and a small reduction in exacerbations [38].
- The Lung Health II Study showed that triamcinolone 600 μg twice daily had no effect on the decline in lung function over 3.5 years in patients with moderate COPD. The study also demonstrated a reduction in bone density in the steroid-treated group [39].

Side effects

The place of inhaled corticosteroids in the management of COPD remains uncertain after these studies. Any benefit is slight and must be weighed against the risk of side effects. Patients with COPD are at particular risk of systemic effects of inhaled corticosteroids (osteoporosis, cataracts, skin bruising, glaucoma) as they are elderly, immobile and often have a poor diet. Patients with COPD are commonly given high doses of inhaled corticosteroids, which have little obvious clinical benefit. In view of the adverse risk–benefit ratio this cannot be recommended.

Corticosteroids in acute exacerbations

There is clear evidence that systemic corticosteroids are useful in acute exacerbations of COPD and improve the rate of recovery, although this effect is relatively small [40–42]. Their mechanism of action in acute exacerbations in contrast to their inefficacy in controlling chronic stable COPD is unexplained. It is possible that corticosteroids reduce airway oedema or that there is a different pattern of inflammation in exacerbations which is corticosteroid-sensitive. Thus, in acute exacerbations an increase in the number of eosinophils has been reported and these cells are potently suppressed by corticosteroids [43]. As corticosteroids are useful in the acute management of exacerbations of COPD, inhaled corticosteroids have been assessed in the prevention of acute exacerbations. In a recent study, high-dose fluticasone propionate was found to have a small protective effect against severe exacerbations [44] (*see* Figure 3.6).

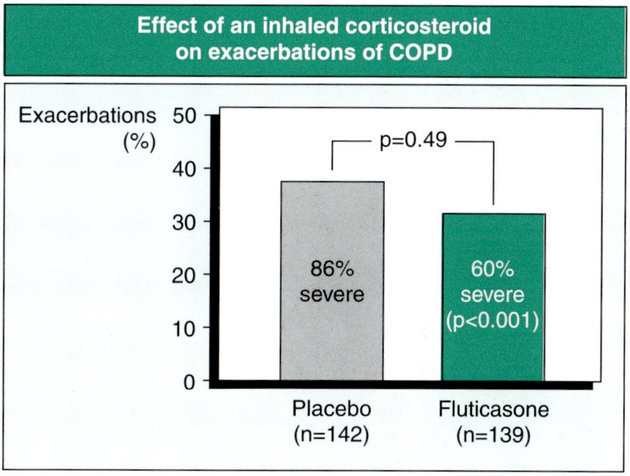

Figure 3.6. Fluticasone propionate (500 μg twice daily) has a small effect in reducing the number and severity of acute exacerbations. Adapted from [45]. © American Lung Association.

Recommended use of inhaled corticosteroids

Inhaled corticosteroids do not alter the progression of COPD, probably because the underlying inflammatory process is steroid-resistant. They have a small protective effect against exacerbations in patients with severe COPD, but this is no more than seen with bronchodilators and has to be offset against the cost of high doses of inhaled corticosteroids and the risk of side effects in a susceptible population. Inhaled corticosteroids should therefore only be recommended in those patients who have concomitant asthma, as demonstrated by a large bronchodilator response or a clear response to oral corticosteroids [45].

Cromones

Sodium cromoglycate and nedocromil sodium have no role in the management of COPD [46].

Antileukotrienes

Cysteinyl-leukotriene antagonists, such as montelukast and zafirlukast, have no place in the management of COPD because these mediators are not involved in the disease process. LTB_4 is not blocked by these drugs but its synthesis may be inhibited by 5-lipoxygenase inhibitors, such as zileuton. However, no trials have yet demonstrated any benefit of these drugs, which are not available in most countries.

Mucolytics

Because mucus hypersecretion is a prominent feature of chronic bronchitis, various mucolytic therapies have been used to increase the ease of mucus expectoration, in the belief that this will improve lung function.

- *Stopping smoking* is the most effective way to reduce mucus hypersecretion.
- *Anticholinergics* may decrease mucus hypersecretion.
- *β_2-Agonists* and *theophylline* may improve mucus clearance.
- *Steam inhalation* (with or without aromatics) may provide symptomatic relief, but there is no evidence that it improves lung function or long-term symptom control.
- Several drugs, such as *carbocisteine, bromhexol* and *ambroxol,* reduce mucus viscosity *in vitro*, but there is little evidence from controlled trials that they improve lung function in patients with COPD, and cannot be recommended as routine therapy.
- Expectorants, such as *guanifeniesin* and *potassium iodide,* similarly have no proven beneficial effects.
- *Recombinant human DNAse* (alfadornase, Pulmozyme) has beneficial effects in some patients with cystic fibrosis, but its role in COPD is not yet clear. Until there is clear evidence of benefit in COPD it should not be used in view of its high cost.

Antioxidants

Since oxidant damage may be critical in the pathophysiology of COPD, antioxidant therapy is logical. N-acetyl cysteine was originally developed as a mucolytic, but has well documented anti-oxidant effects. Controlled trials have demonstrated that it reduces the frequency and severity of acute exacerbations of COPD [47] and in an open study significantly reduced the rate of decline in lung function [48]. It may therefore be useful in long-term management of COPD, but is not currently available on prescription in the UK. A recent meta-analysis demonstrated a beneficial effect of N-acetyl cysteine in reducing exacerbations of COPD by approximately 25% [49,50].

Vaccines

Influenza vaccine is usually recommended as patients with COPD are subject to severe exacerbations with this infection and there is evidence for a reduction in acute exacerbations and hospital admissions [51]. There is now convincing evidence that influenza vaccination is cost effective in elderly people and should be more so in patients with COPD [52]. Influenza vaccination should be given every autumn. Polyvalent pneumococcal vaccine is used in many countries to protect against the development of pneumococcal lung infections [53]. Pneumococcal vaccination is cost-effective in reducing infective exacerbations in COPD [54]. OM85-BV (Broncho-Vaxom) is a mixture of bacterial products that activate macrophage function (the advantage of which is obscure!). There is some evidence that it may reduce the severity of acute exacerbations, but it cannot be recommended as a routine treatment [55].

Neuraminidase inhibitors

Inhibitors of neuraminidase, such as zanamivir (inhaled) and oseltamivir (oral) speed the recovery from influenza and may protect against its development [56,57]. However, no specific trials have been conducted in patients with COPD, and it is not yet certain whether this treatment is cost-effective.

Treatment of dyspnoea

Breathlessness is a problem in many patients, particularly 'pink puffers'. Several drugs, including nebulized opiates, slow-release morphine, dihydrocodeine and benzodiazepines, may reduce the sensation of dyspnoea but the reduction in ventilatory drive is potentially dangerous and these drugs should be avoided, particularly during exacerbations [58].

Respiratory stimulants

There is no role for respiratory stimulants, such as doxapram or almitrine, in the long-term management of COPD, since there is no evidence that central ventilatory drive is impaired. Ventilation is limited by mechanical rather than neurophysiological factors. However, doxapram may be indicated in the management of an acute exacerbation of COPD if there is hypercapnia and hypoventilation in order to tide the patient over 24–36 hours until the underlying cause (eg, infection) is controlled. However, it is likely that the use of doxapram in this situation will decline as nasal intermittent positive pressure ventilation (NIPPV) becomes more widely available.

Antitussives

Cough is often a troublesome symptom of COPD, but may have a protective effect in clearing secretions. The regular use of antitussives is therefore not recommended as treatment in COPD [59].

References

1. Nisar M, Earis JE, Pearson MG *et al.* **Acute bronchodilator trials in chronic obstructive pulmonary disease.** *Am Rev Respir Dis* 1992; **146**:555–559.

2. O'Donnell DE, Lam M, Webb KA. **Measurement of symptoms, lung hyperinflation, and endurance during exercise in chronic obstructive pulmonary disease.** *Am J Respir Crit Care Med* 1998; **158**:1557–1565.

3. Belman MJ, Botnick WC, Shin JW. **Inhaled bronchodilators reduce dynamic hyperinflation during exercise in patients with chronic obstructive pulmonary disease.** *Am J Respir Crit Care Med* 1996; **153**:967–975.

4. Gross NJ. **Anticholinergic bronchodilators.** In: *Asthma: Basic Mechanisms and Clinical Management, 3rd edition.* Edited by PJ Barnes, IW Rodger and NC Thomson. London: Academic Press, 1998;555–566.

5. Rennard SI, Serby CW, Ghafouri M *et al.* **Extended therapy with ipratropium is associated with improved lung function in patients with COPD. A retrospective analysis of data from seven clinical trials.** *Chest* 1996; **110**:62–70.

6. Tamaoki J, Chiyotani A, Tagaya E *et al.* **Effect of long-term treatment with oxitropium bromide on airway secretion in chronic bronchitis and diffuse panbronchiolitis.** *Thorax* 1994; **49**:545–548.

7. Combivent Inhalation Aerosol Study Group. **In chronic obstructive pulmonary disease, a combination of ipratropium and albuterol is more effective than either agent alone. An 85-day multicenter trial.** *Chest* 1994; **105**:1411–1419.

8. Dowling RB, Johnson M, Cole PJ *et al.* **Effect of salmeterol on *Haemophilus influenzae* infection of respiratory mucosa *in vitro*.** *Eur Respir J* 1998; **11**:86–90.

9. Suzuki S, Watanuki Y, Yoshiike Y *et al.* **Effects of fenoterol on ventilatory response to hypercapnia and hypoxia in patients with chronic obstructive pulmonary disease.** *Thorax* 1997; **52**:125–129.

10. Appleton S, Smith B, Veale A *et al.* **Long-acting β_2-agonists for chronic obstructive pulmonary disease.** *Cochrane Database Syst Rev* 2000; **2**:CD001104: CD001104

11. Jones PW, Bosh TK. **Quality of life changes in COPD patients treated with salmeterol.** *Am J Respir Crit Care Med* 1997; **155**:1283–1289.

12. Cazzola M, Matera MG, Di Perna F *et al.* **A comparison of bronchodilating effects of salmeterol and oxitropium bromide in stable chronic obstructive pulmonary disease.** *Respir Med* 1998; **92**:354–357.

13. McDonald CF, Pierce RJ, Thompson PJ *et al.* **Comparison of oral bambuterol and terbutaline in elderly patients with chronic reversible airflow obstruction.** *J Asthma* 1997; **34**:53–59.

14. Crompton GK, Ayres JG, Basran G *et al.* **Comparison of oral bambuterol and inhaled salmeterol in patients with symptomatic asthma and using inhaled corticosteroids.** *Am J Respir Crit Care Med* 1999; **159**:824–828.

15. Wallaert B, Brun P, Ostinelli J *et al.* **A comparison of two long-acting beta-agonists, oral bambuterol and inhaled salmeterol, in the treatment of moderate to severe asthmatic patients with nocturnal symptoms. The French Bambuterol Study Group.** *Respir Med* 1999; **93**:33–38.

16. Chrystyn H, Mulley BA, Peake MD. **Dose–response relation to oral theophylline in severe chronic obstructive airway disease.** *BMJ* 1988; **297**:1506–1510.

17. Culpitt S, Maziak W, Loukides S *et al.* **Effect of theophylline on induced sputum inflammatory indices in COPD patients [Abstract].** *Am J Respir Crit Care Med* 1997; **157**:A797.

18. ZuWallack RL, Mahler DA, Reilly D *et al.* **Salmeterol plus theophylline combination therapy in the treatment of COPD.** *Chest* 2001; **119**:1661–1670.

19. Seemungal T, Harper-Owen R, Bhowmik A *et al.* **Detection of rhinoviruses in induced sputum at exacerbations of chronic obstructive pulmonary disease.** *Eur Respir J* 2000; **16**:677–683.

20. Saint S, Bent S, Vittinghoff E *et al.* **Antibiotics in chronic obstructive pulmonary disease exacerbations. A meta-analysis.** *JAMA* 1995; **273**:957–960.

21. Tarpy SP, Celli B. **Long-term oxygen therapy.** *N Engl J Med* 1995; **333**:710–714.

22. Restrick LJ, Paul EA, Braid GM *et al.* **Assessment and follow-up of patients prescribed long-term oxygen treatment.** *Thorax* 1993; **48**:708–713.

23. Wedzicha JA. **Domiciliary oxygen therapy services: clinical guidelines and advice for prescribers. Summary of a report of the Royal College of Physicians.** *J R Coll Physicians Lond* 1999; **33**:445–447.

24. Anonymous. **Continuous or nocturnal oxygen therapy in hypoxemic chronic obstructive lung disease: a clinical trial. Nocturnal Oxygen Therapy Trial Group.** *Ann Intern Med* 1980; **93**:391–398.

25. Anonymous. **Long term domiciliary oxygen therapy in chronic hypoxic cor pulmonale complicating chronic bronchitis and emphysema. Report of the Medical Research Council Working Party.** *Lancet* 1981; **1**:681–686.

26. Georgopoulos D, Anthonisen NR. **Continuous oxygen therapy for the chronically hypoxemic patient.** *Annu Rev Med* 1990; **41**:223–230.

27. Crockett AJ, Moss JR, Cranston JM *et al*. **Domicilary oxygen for chronic obstructive pulmonary disease.** *Cochrane Database Syst Rev* 2000; CD001744.

28. Department of Health. *Domiciliary Oxygen Therapy Service.* Drug tarriff 1990, Part X, HMSO.

29. Walshaw MJ, Lim R, Evans CC *et al*. **Prescription of oxygen concentrators for long-term oxygen treatment: reassessment in one district.** *BMJ* 1988; **297**:1030–1032.

30. McEvoy CE, Niewoehner DE. **Adverse effects of corticosteroid therapy for COPD. A critical review.** *Chest* 1997; **111**:732–743.

31. Kwon OJ, Au BT, Collins PD *et al*. **Tumor necrosis factor-induced interleukin 8 expression in cultured human epithelial cells.** *Am J Physiol* 1994; **11**:L398–L405.

32. Abbinante-Nissen JM, Simpson LG, Leikauf GD. **Corticosteroids increase secretory leucocyte protease inhibitor transcript levels in airway epithelial cells.** *Am J Physiol* 1995; **12**:L601–L606.

33. Keatings VM, Jatakanon A, Worsdell YM *et al*. **Effects of inhaled and oral glucocorticoids on inflammatory indices in asthma and COPD.** *Am J Respir Crit Care Med* 1997; **155**:542–548.

34. Culpitt SV, Nightingale JA, Barnes PJ. **Effect of high dose inhaled steroid on cells, cytokines and proteases in induced sputum in chronic obstructive pulmonary disease.** *Am J Respir Crit Care Med* 1999; **160**:1635–1639.

35. Ito K, Lim S, Caramori G *et al*. **Cigarette smoking reduces histone deacetylase 2 expression, enhances cytokine expression and inhibits glucocorticoid actions in alveolar macrophages.** *FASEB J* 2001; **15**:1100–1102.

36. Vestbo J, Sorensen T, Lange P *et al*. **Long-term effect of inhaled budesonide in mild and moderate chronic obstructive pulmonary disease: a randomized controlled trial.** *Lancet* 1999; **353**:1819–1823.

37. Pauwels RA, Lofdahl CG, Laitinen LA *et al*. **Long-term treatment with inhaled budesonide in persons with mild chronic obstructive pulmonary disease who continue smoking.** *N Engl J Med* 1999; **340**:1948–1953.

38. Burge PS, Calverley PMA, Jones PW *et al*. **Randomised, double-blind, placebo-controlled study of fluticasone propionate in patients with moderate to severe chronic obstructive pulmonary disease, the ISOLDE trial.** *BMJ* 2000; **320**:1297–1303.

39. Lung Health Study Research Group. **Effect of inhaled triamcinolone on the decline in pulmonary function in chronic obstructive pulmonary disease.** *N Engl J Med* 2000; **343**:1902–1909.

40. Thompson WH, Nielson CP, Carvalho P *et al*. **Controlled trial of oral prednisone in outpatients with acute COPD exacerbation.** *Am J Respir Crit Care Med* 1996; **154**:407–412.

41. Davies L, Angus RM, Calverley PM. **Oral corticosteroids in patients admitted to hospital with exacerbations of chronic obstructive pulmonary disease: a prospective randomised controlled trial.** *Lancet* 1999; **354**:456–460.

42. Niewoehner DE, Erbland ML, Deupree RH *et al*. **Effect of systemic glucocorticoids on exacerbations of chronic obstructive pulmonary disease.** *N Engl J Med* 1999; **340**:1941–1947.

43. Saetta M, Distefano A, Maestrelli P *et al*. **Airway eosinophilia in chronic bronchitis during exacerbations.** *Am J Respir Crit Care Med* 1994; **150**:1646–1652.

44. Paggiaro PL, Dahle R, Bakran I *et al*. **Multicentre randomised placebo-controlled trial of inhaled fluticasone propionate in patients with chronic obstructive pulmonary disease.** *Lancet* 1998; **351**:773–780.

45. Barnes PJ. **Inhaled corticosteroids are not helpful in chronic obstructive pulmonary disease.** *Am J Respir Crit Care Med* 2000; **161**:342–344.

46. de Jong JW, Postma DS, Van der Mark TW *et al*. **Effects of nedocromil sodium in the treatment of non-allergic subjects with chronic obstructive pulmonary disease.** *Thorax* 1994; **49**:1022–1024.

47. Boman G, Backer U, Larsson S *et al*. **Oral acetylcysteine reduces exacerbation rate in chronic bronchitis: report of a trial organized by the Swedish Society for Pulmonary Diseases.** *Eur J Respir Dis* 1983; **64**:405–415.

48. Lundback B, Lindstrom M, Jonsson E *et al.* **Effect of N-acetylcysteine on the decline in lung function in patients with COPD.** *Eur Respir J* 1995; **5**(Suppl 15):895.

49. Grandjean EM, Berthet P, Ruffmann R *et al.* **Efficacy of oral long-term N-acetylcysteine in chronic bronchopulmonary disease: a meta-analysis of published double-blind, placebo-controlled clinical trials.** *Clin Ther* 2000; **22**:209–221.

50. Poole PJ, Black PN. **Oral mucolytic drugs for exacerbations of chronic obstructive pulmonary disease: systematic review.** *BMJ* 2001; **322**:1271–1274.

51. Poole PJ, Chacko E, Wood-Baker RW *et al.* **Influenza vaccine for patients with chronic obstructive pulmonary disease (Cochrane Review).** *Cochrane Database Syst Rev* 2000; CD002733.

52. Nichol KL, Baken L, Wuorenma J *et al.* **The health and economic benefits associated with pneumococcal vaccination of elderly persons with chronic lung disease.** *Arch Intern Med* 1999; **159**:2437–2442.

53. Fedson DS, Shapiro ED, LaForce FM *et al.* **Pneumococcal vaccine after 15 years of use. Another view.** *Arch Intern Med* 1994; **154**:2531–2535.

54. Nichol KL, Baken L, Wuorenma J *et al.* **The health and economic benefits associated with pneumococcal vaccination of elderly persons with chronic lung disease.** *Arch Intern Med* 1999; **159**:2437–2442.

55. Collet JP, Shapiro P, Ernst P *et al.* **Effects of an immunostimulating agent on acute exacerbations and hospitalizations in patients with chronic obstructive pulmonary disease. The PARI-IS Study Steering Committee and Research Group. Prevention of Acute Respiratory Infection by an Immunostimulant.** *Am J Respir Crit Care Med* 1997; **156**:1719–1724.

56. Dunn CJ, Goa KL. **Zanamivir: a review of its use in influenza.** *Drugs* 1999; **58**:761–784.

57. Bardsley-Elliot A, Noble S. **Oseltamivir.** *Drugs* 1999; **58**:851–860.

57. Poole PJ, Veale AG, Black PN. **The effect of sustained-release morphine on breathlessness and quality of life in severe chronic obstructive pulmonary disease.** *Am J Respir Crit Care Med* 1998; **157**:1877–1880.

59. Irwin RS, Boulet LP, Cloutier MM *et al.* **Managing cough as a defense mechanism and as a symptom. A consensus panel report of the American College of Chest Physicians.** *Chest* 1998; **114**:133S–1381S.

Chapter 4

Management of COPD

Managing COPD depends upon evaluating the severity of the disorder, providing appropriate treatment and evaluating the response — usually on a long-term basis over many years. Guidelines for the management of COPD have been formulated in several counties [1–3] and recently the international GOLD guidelines have been introduced [4].

Key elements in the management of COPD are:

- assessment and monitoring of disease;
- reduction or avoidance of risk factors;
- management of stable COPD; and
- management and prevention of exacerbations.

Goals of treatment

Management should be designed to:

- prevent disease progression;
- relieve symptoms;
- improve exercise tolerance;
- improve health status;
- prevent and treat exacerbations;
- prevent and treat complications;
- reduce mortality; and
- avoid or minimize side effects of therapy in achieving these aims.

Management usually involves:

- cessation of smoking;
- bronchodilator therapy;
- supplementary oxygen when needed;
- treatment of heart failure;
- treatment of respiratory failure, possibly by mechanical ventilation;
- pulmonary rehabilitation;
- possible palliative surgery for emphysema; and
- early detection and treatment of pulmonary malignancy.

Assessment

Clinical assessment

- Quality of life, ability to work or engage in normal social activities.
- Frequency of cough and sputum production.

- Quantity and quality of sputum.
- Degree of exercise limitation.
- Breathlessness at rest.
- Sleep disturbance.
- Frequency of acute exacerbations of COPD.
- Appearance of signs of heart failure — cor pulmonale.

Radiological assessment

- Plain chest radiograph when any significant clinical change occurs; useful to exclude alternative diagnoses.
- CT scan of chest if there is any suspicion of malignancy and if surgical treatment is contemplated.
- Special radiological techniques if needed (spiral CT, angiography etc.).

Physiological assessment

- Spirometry (± bronchodilator response) at every clinic visit and at least twice/year.
- Pulse oximetry whenever deterioration is suspected.
- Arterial blood gas assessment is important in severe disease and if respiratory failure is suspected.
- Full lung function tests including measurement of lung volumes, blood gases and carbon monoxide transfer factor if major clinical change occurs or if surgery is contemplated.
- Sleep study if there is suspicion of significant hypoxia during sleep or other sleep disturbances.
- Simple exercise test — six-minute walk, shuttle test or step test — may be useful periodically.

Cardiac assessment

- Indicated periodically to detect early signs of right heart failure (cor pulmonale) so that attempts can be made to step up treatment and improve oxygenation.
- ECG should be performed to detect coexisting ischaemic heart disease, but is relatively insensitive in detecting right ventricular hypertrophy, particularly with hyperinflation.
- Echocardiography is indicated to provide better information on right ventricular function and pulmonary artery pressure in patients with suspected cor pulmonale.

Other investigations

- Sputum examination is not usually helpful but may give important information in patients who fail to respond to usual antibiotics for acute exacerbation.

- Biochemical/haematological investigations as indicated by clinical condition such as diuretic therapy, suspicion of polycythaemia and chronic hypoxia, or if α_1-antitrypsin deficiency is suspected.
- Fibreoptic bronchoscopy should be used as in any other patient when there is the suspicion of malignancy.

Management of stable COPD

Guidelines for COPD propose a logical approach to management based on best available evidence, although there is still relatively little evidence from controlled trials to dictate the optimal therapy (*see* Figures 4.1 and 4.2).

Stopping smoking

Stopping smoking is the single most beneficial management strategy and is the only intervention that reduces the accelerated decline in lung function (*see* Figure 4.3) [5].

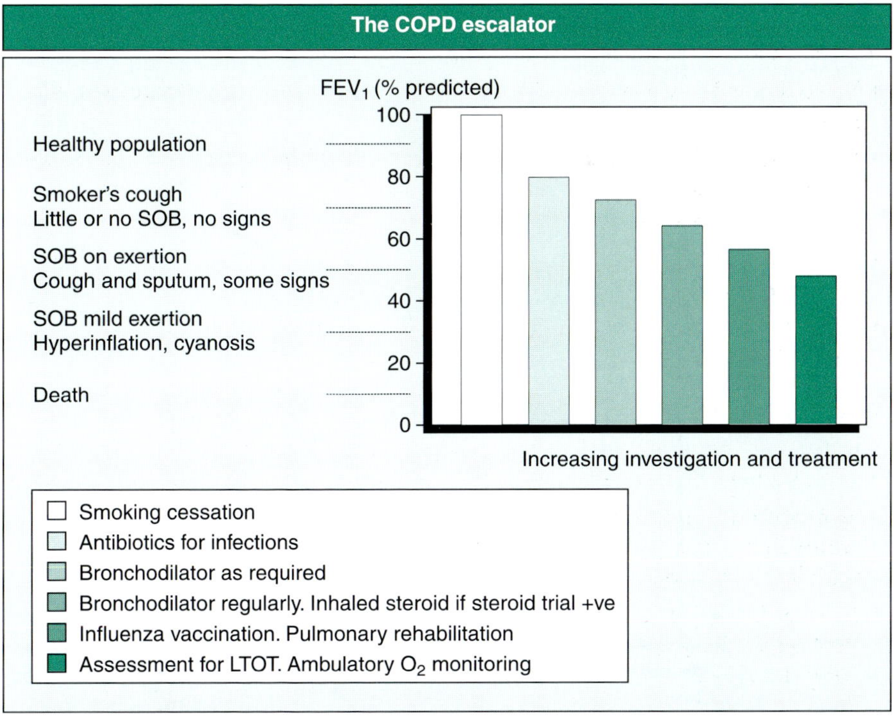

Figure 4.1. As the disease progresses there is an increasing need for investigation and treatment. COPD, chronic obstructive pulmonary disease; SOB, shortness of breath; LTOT, long-term oxygen therapy. Adapted from [3]. © BMJ Publishing Group.

Management of COPD

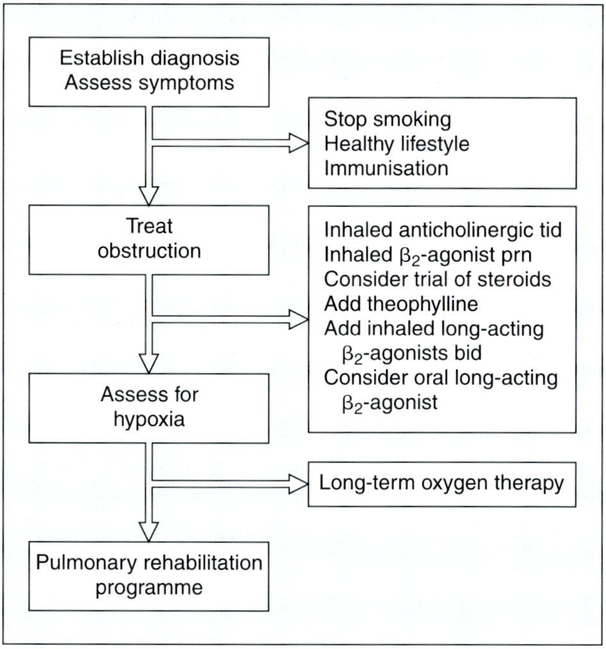

Figure 4.2. Summary of progressive treatment approaches. COPD, chronic obstructive pulmonary disease; tid, three times daily; prn, as required; bid, twice daily.

Impact of smoking cessation on decline in lung function

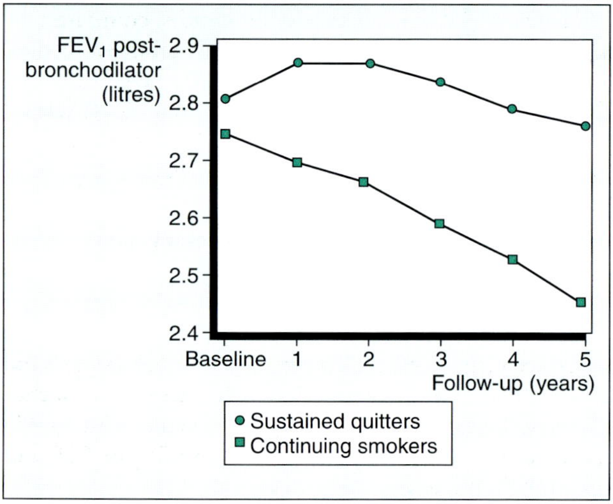

Figure 4.3. Smoking cessation reduces the rate of decline of lung function in patients with chronic obstructive pulmonary disease (COPD).

It is important even in patients with severe disease. Nicotine addiction is the major problem and treatment should be directed at dealing with this addictive state. The major approaches involve behavioural approaches and nicotine replacement therapy, but the overall rates of quitting are small (5–15%) [6]. Abrupt quitting is more successful than gradual reduction, but even after an intensive smoking cessation programme, over 75% of smokers are still smoking one year later. There are several ways to encourage smoking cessation [6].

- *Psychological counselling* and *smoking reduction clinics* may be useful (addresses in UK available from Quitline: 0207 487 3000). Advice from doctors, structured interventions from nurses, and individual and group counselling are all effective [6].
- *Group therapy* may help some patients.
- *Nicotine replacement therapy* doubles long-term (6–12 months) abstinence rates [7]. Several forms are available, all of which have some effect [8]:
  - nicotine chewing gum is the most widely used but the least effective;
  - nicotine skin patches are somewhat more successful;
  - nasal nicotine spray has a greater success rate because it gives a more rapid rise in plasma nicotine concentrations; and
  - nicotine inhaler is the most successful form because it most closely mimics the intake of nicotine in a cigarette.
- *Hypnosis* and *acupuncture* may be helpful in some patients but controlled trials have demonstrated that they are ineffective [6].
- *Clonidine*, an α_2-adrenergic agonist has some efficacy, but side effects (especially sedation) are common, so it is not recommended.
- *Bupropion* is an atypical antidepressant that helps with smoking cessation. Its mechanism of action may involve inhibition of noradrenaline and dopamine uptake, rather than its antidepressant effect. Bupropion is given as a short course (6–9 weeks) and provides sustained quit rates of 18% at 12 months, compared with 10% with nicotine skin patches and 6% with placebo [9]. Combined bupropion and nicotine skin patch yielded a quit rate of 22%, which is not significantly better than the rate with bupropion alone. Results in patients with COPD are similar [10]. Bupropion is well tolerated apart from its attendant sleeplessness, but epileptic fits occur in approximately 0.1% of patients, predominantly those with previous epilepsy [11].
- *Other antidepressants*, such as fluoxetine and tricyclic antidepressants and anxiolytics are unhelpful in smoking cessation [12].

Bronchodilator treatment

The use of bronchodilators to reduce symptoms and increase exercise tolerance is the cornerstone of management of COPD. There is no evidence that chronic bronchodilator treatment alters the natural history of COPD [13]. In patients with COPD symptomatic improvement may not be reflected by an increase in FEV_1 or PEF and may be due to other actions of bronchodilators:

- reduction in pulmonary hyperinflation due to an effect on peripheral airways which makes breathing more comfortable and reduces the work of breathing and the sensation of dyspnoea;
- increase in exercise tolerance;
- changes in mucociliary clearance; and
- improvement in respiratory muscle function, although this is unlikely at the doses of drugs used clinically.

The choice of bronchodilator may depend on individual patients. Anticholinergics appear to be more effective bronchodilators than β_2-agonists and should be given on a regular basis (eg, ipratropium bromide 40–80 μg three times daily or oxitropium bromide 200 mg three times daily). Short acting β_2-agonists (eg, salbutamol 200 μg or terbutaline 500 μg) should be used as additional treatments as required for symptom control. Inhaled long-acting β_2-agonists (salmeterol 50 μg twice daily or formoterol 12–24 μg twice daily) may be useful additional bronchodilators and are additive with anticholinergics [14]. Slow-release theophylline is also useful and may have particular value in reducing hyperinflation by acting on peripheral airways [15].

Combination bronchodilator inhalers with an anticholinergic and a short-acting β_2-agonist, such as Combivent (ipratropium bromide and salbutamol) are a convenient way of giving bronchodilators and are preferred by patients [16].

Delivery systems

Anticholinergics and β_2-agonists are best given by MDI or DPI. In an evaluation of how well patients with COPD used inhaler devices, 76% of patients made important errors with MDIs, whereas only 40% made errors with DPIs [17]. A large volume spacer can be helpful in increasing delivery to the lungs in patients with more severe airways obstruction.

Home nebulizers

Home nebulizers should be reserved for the patients with the most severe airflow obstruction when other forms of inhaler have failed [18]. Nebulized bronchodilator therapy is much more expensive than MDIs or DPIs. Any patient who is prescribed a home nebulizer should be assessed by a specialist.

Non-bronchodilator drug treatments

Inhaled corticosteroids

Approximately 10% of patients with COPD show some improvement with a trial of oral corticosteroids and it is best to regard these patients as having coexisting asthma and to treat them as if they have asthma. For the remainder of patients there is little evidence that inhaled corticosteroids are beneficial in the long-term management of COPD, as discussed in Chapter 3. Because high dose inhaled corticosteroids are likely to have systemic side effects in this group of patients they should not be used. They are also relatively expensive.

Long-term oxygen therapy

LTOT can be prescribed by the general practitioner in England and Wales, but all patients should be assessed by a specialist. Arterial blood gas measurements should be taken when the patient is clinically stable and on optimal therapy on at least two occasions three weeks apart. LTOT should be prescribed for patients with a PaO_2 of less than 7.3 kPa (<55 mmHg) with or without hypercapnia and with an FEV_1 of less than 1.5 litres. LTOT should also be considered if PaO_2 is 7.3–8.0 kPa (55–60 mmHg) and there is evidence of pulmonary hypertension, peripheral oedema or nocturnal hypoxaemia. Blood gas measurements should be made when patients are on LTOT to ensure that PaO_2 is more than 8.0 kPa (>60 mmHg) without a rise in $PaCO_2$. LTOT should be give for at least 15 hours a day to achieve benefit. This therapy is most efficiently provided by an oxygen concentrator and nasal prongs set at a flow of 2–4 l/min. Patients on LTOT should be reassessed regularly. LTOT can improve quality of life [19].

Ambulatory oxygen

Ambulatory oxygen may improve exercise tolerance and breathlessness in patients with severe COPD. Improvement is related to the degree of arterial oxygen desaturation on exercise [20]. Prescription of ambulatory oxygen should be based on documented desaturation on a standard walking test (>4% fall in saturation below 90%). Portable cylinders provide two hours of oxygen at 2 l/min.

Mucolytic therapy

Mucolytic therapies have not proved to be very effective, although there is some evidence that N-acetyl cysteine is beneficial in acute exacerbations and in long-term therapy; this is probably because of its antioxidant effect rather than as a mucolytic therapy.

Antibiotics

There is no evidence that prophylactic antibiotics reduce the incidence or severity of infective exacerbations of COPD. However, antibiotics (*see* Chapter 3) should be started at the first sign of an exacerbation.

Antidepressants

Depression is very common, particularly in severe COPD [21]. Antidepressants may be indicated in selected patients.

Non-pharmacological treatments

Several non-pharmacological approaches have also been used in the management of COPD and may form part of a comprehensive rehabilitation programme.

Exercise

Exercise training to improve cardio-respiratory function may be helpful; the type of exercise does not appear to be important, and aerobic exercise or upper limb exercises are equally effective [22,23]. Respiratory muscle training using resistive inspiratory loading may reduce breathlessness, but a meta-analysis of controlled studies of respiratory muscle training alone has provided no evidence of overall benefit [24]. Controlled breathing techniques, such as pursed-lip breathing and diaphragmatic breathing, result in reduced dyspnoea, particularly in patients with hyperventilation.

Nutrition

Nutrition is important in patients with COPD and many patients are malnourished and underweight. Reduced fat-free mass is associated with a poor prognosis [25].

Obese patients should lose weight, particularly if there are sleep disturbances. Antioxidant vitamin supplements are also indicated. However, there are no controlled trials to document the value of improved nutrition on COPD and attempts to correct nutritional deficiency by food supplementation alone have not been successful [26].

Pulmonary rehabilitation

Rehabilitation concerns prevention of deconditioning and allowing the patient to cope with his/her disease. Pulmonary rehabilitation includes physical exercise training and disease education, with psychological and social support. Rehabilitation programmes are successful in prospective randomized trials in terms of increased performance and quality of life [27–29]. Patients with moderate to severe COPD should be considered for pulmonary rehabilitation programmes, which include educational advice and physiotherapy. Most rehabilitation programmes are based on hospital outpatients. The optimal duration and frequency of rehabilitation programmes is not known. Resources in the UK are currently limited.

Disease education

Disease education and psychological support may reduce exercise-induced dyspnoea.

Referral to hospital

Referral to a respiratory physician is useful to: establish the diagnosis and differentiate from asthma; exclude other pathology, including malignancy; reinforce the need to stop smoking; and optimize therapy.

Referral is indicated in particular patients: early onset of disease or family history of α_1-antitrypsin deficiency; signs of cor pulmonale; assessment of LTOT or nebulizer therapy; those with a rapid decline in lung function (>100 ml/year); and those with frequent infections to exclude bronchiectasis.

Follow-up assessment

Regular follow-up is important in order to: assess disease progression with measurement of FEV_1; supervise smoking cessation; assess the benefits of drug treatment; and assess clinical status in severe COPD to detect signs of cor pulmonale, need for LTOT and home nebulizers.

Treatment of acute exacerbations

Clinical features

Acute exacerbations of COPD present as a worsening of the previous stable situation. They may be due to bacterial or viral infections, or to non-infective causes (*see* Figure 4.4). The features are an increase in cough and sputum volume; increase in breathlessness ± wheeze; increase in hypoxia; peripheral oedema; and increase in airways obstruction measured by spirometry.

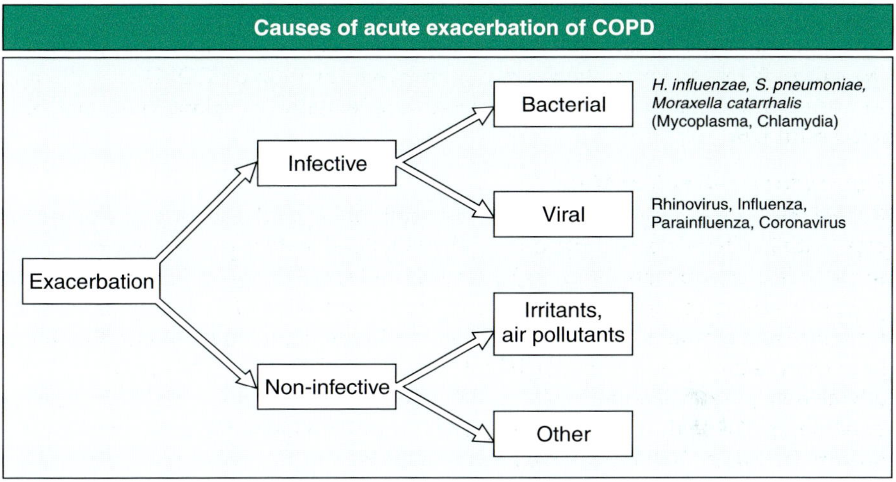

Figure 4.4. Acute exacerbations of chronic obstructive pulmonary disease (COPD) may be from bacterial or viral infection, or from non-infective causes.

Differential diagnosis

- Pneumonia.
- Pulmonary embolism.
- Spontaneous pneumothorax.
- Left ventricular failure/pulmonary oedema.
- Lung cancer.
- Upper airway obstruction.

Assessment

Most patients can be managed at home, but hospital management should be considered in most cases of: inability to cope at home, living alone; severe breathlessness; cyanosis; worsening peripheral oedema; and acute confusion.

Management in general practice

- Start a course of antibiotics. Antibiotics are effective only if sputum is purulent, there is an increase in volume and there is increased breathlessness. Not all infective exacerbations are due to bacteria.
- Increase (or begin) inhaled β_2-agonist and anticholinergic bronchodilator — give three to four times daily by MDI and spacer or jet nebulizer.
- Oral steroids (prednisolone 30 mg daily for one week) are indicated if this has previously been shown to improve lung function or airflow obstruction has not responded to increased doses of bronchodilator.
- Follow up to ensure that the patient has improved.

Management in hospital

Evidence on optimal management of acute exacerbations of COPD is relatively patchy [30].

- Arterial blood gases should be measured and a chest radiograph arranged.
- Oxygen (24 or 28% via Venturi mask) should be given to achieve a PaO_2 of at least 6.6 kPa (50 mmHg) without a fall in pH to less than 7.26 (indicating an acute change). Check blood gases within one hour of starting oxygen therapy. Oxygen saturation by pulse oximetry may be used to monitor response providing $PaCO_2$ and pH are normal.
- Bronchodilators (ipratropium bromide 0.25–0.5 mg plus salbutamol 2.5–5 mg) should be given by nebulization four to six hourly and continued for 24–48 hours. If no response intravenous aminophylline should be added (0.5 mg/kg/h) [31].
- Antibiotics should be started if indicated (as above). In severe exacerbations sputum culture should be done for antibiotic sensitivity.
- Oral corticosteroids are indicated for a severe exacerbation (prednisolone 30 mg daily for 7–14 days). A course of oral steroids administered during the first 72 hours speeds recovery and reduces duration of hospital stay. However, side effects may be a problem and there is no evidence that there is any long-term benefit [32–34].
- Diuretics are indicated if there is peripheral oedema.
- Chest physiotherapy may be useful (but there is no evidence from controlled studies that it improves recovery).

Discharge from hospital

- Record FEV_1 before discharge.
- Arterial blood gases checked in patients with a low PaO_2 on admission or with respiratory failure.
- Switch nebulized bronchodilators to MDI or DPI at least 24 hours before discharge.
- Check inhaler technique.
- Review all medication.
- Check that patient understands how to use medication.
- Assess home needs.
- Give follow-up appointment four to six weeks after discharge.

Respiratory failure

Chronic respiratory failure

Clinical features

- Often develops insidiously and may be undetected in COPD.
- Carbon dioxide retention with persistently elevated arterial PCO_2 ($PaCO_2$): hypercapnic respiratory failure.

- Metabolic compensation with elevated plasma bicarbonate and relatively normal pH.
- Hypoxia which may be disproportionate to elevated $PaCO_2$ because of concomitant V/Q mismatching in the lungs.
- May become worse during sleep.
- May be associated with mental confusion if severe.
- Often leads to cor pulmonale.
- Patients may underventilate when given oxygen because ventilation is largely driven by hypoxia.

Management

The management of chronic respiratory failure is basically same as the management of COPD: treat cor pulmonale if present; follow oxygen saturation and check $PaCO_2$ periodically. Home NIPPV via nasal masks has recently been shown to be very effective in patients with hypercapnic respiratory failure, but it is available only in a few centres and is still being assessed [35,36]. Respiratory stimulants (doxapram, almitrine) are not indicated because ventilatory drive is already maximal.

Acute respiratory failure

Clinical features

- Often develops on basis of chronic respiratory failure due to infection or some other complication such as pulmonary embolism or pulmonary artery thrombosis.
- Patient becomes more hypoxic with cyanosis.
- Underventilation causes rising $PaCO_2$ and falling pH.
- Patient becomes confused and drowsy.
- Patient becomes tired and ventilation deteriorates further.
- Consciousness may be lost and respiratory arrest ensues.

Management

- First priority — ensure adequate but not excessive oxygenation — arterial saturation about 85–90%.
- Treat COPD with bronchodilators, physiotherapy and antibiotics.
- Monitor condition closely, including $PaCO_2$.

Patient improving — continue treatment

Patient deteriorating:

- progressive rise in $PaCO_2$, fatigue and/or confusion;
- start NIPPV if available as this reduces the need for invasive intermittent positive pressure ventilation via endotracheal tube [37,38];
- if NIPPV not available or if patient confused intubate and start IPPV if considered suitable (see below);
- once ventilated effectively sedation may be given to allow patient to rest;

- reduce $PaCO_2$ slowly over 24–48 hours by ventilation to reasonable levels (usually to normal $PaCO_2$ level for patient plus about 5–10 mmHg); and
- when blood gases satisfactory, patient conscious, try extubation or stopping NIPPV and follow clinical state and arterial blood gases.

Patient improving — continue treatment

Patient deteriorating:

- re-institute mechanical ventilation; and
- consider possible need for prolonged home ventilation.

Suitability for IPPV

IPPV is indicated if: a remedial reason for the current deterioration is found (eg, pneumonia); if it is the first episode of respiratory failure; and if the patient has an acceptable quality of life and reasonable level of activity.

IPPV is *not* indicated if there is: previously documented severe COPD which was unresponsive to relevant therapy; quality of life is poor (eg, patient housebound); or there is severe co-existing disease (eg, malignancy, pulmonary oedema).

Cor pulmonale

Cor pulmonale is due to the effect of disease and chronic hypoxia on the pulmonary vasculature.

Clinical features

- Oedema of ankles.
- Elevated jugular venous pressure.
- Prominent pulmonary second heart sound on auscultation (difficult to hear because of overinflation).
- Crackles at lung bases.
- Cardiomegaly on chest radiograph.
- ECG showing P-pulmonale in lead 2 and right ventricular hypertrophy.
- Echocardiography showing enlargement of right ventricle, pulmonary hypertension and sometimes reduced right ventricular ejection fraction.

Management

- Treat COPD with optimum therapy.
- LTOT more than 15 h/day.
- Diuretics to reduce fluid retention.
- Angiotensin converting enzyme (ACE) inhibitors (captopril, enalapril) may be useful.
- Digoxin is only indicated if there is coexistent atrial fibrillation.
- Vasodilators may be hazardous as they lower systemic as well as pulmonary blood pressure.

Surgery

There is a long history of surgery for COPD. Previously used techniques included vagal nerve section and carotid body surgery (to reduce breathlessness), but there was no convincing evidence for benefit. More recently surgical techniques have been successfully applied to more severe emphysema [39].

Lung transplantation

Originally heart–lung transplantation was used in patients with end-stage emphysema, but more recently single lung transplantation (SLT) has become the favoured technique, in view of the difficulty in obtaining donor organs and improvement in lung preservation and anaesthetic management [40]. Availability of donor lungs is severely limited.

Because of problems with residual infection in the remaining lung and of hyperinflation of the existing lung if there is extensive bullous disease, heart–lung transplantation or preferably bilateral sequential SLT is used in patients with these complications.

Patient selection

- Upper age limit of 60 years is usually used.
- Patients with a life expectancy of less than 18 months, or onset of cor pulmonale.
- Recurrent or persistent sepsis and bilateral extensive bullous disease are contraindications to SLT.
- Previous thoracic surgery is a contraindication (haemorrhage).
- Good renal and hepatic function are important.
- Right ventricular failure is not a contraindication.
- Psychological factors and a supportive family are important.
- Criteria for referral for lung transplantation: FEV_1 less than 35% predicted, PaO_2 less than 7.3–8.0 kPa (<55–60 mmHg), $PaCO_2$ more than 6.7 kPa (50 mmHg) and secondary pulmonary hypertension [41].

Complications

- Lung infection (opportunistic infections due to immunosuppression).
- Acute rejection (confirmed by transbronchial biopsy).
- Chronic rejection (obliterative bronchiolitis).

Prognosis

- 10–15% early mortality due to sepsis or diffuse alveolar damage.
- One year survival 70–75%, three year survival 60%.
- Marked improvement in quality of life and lung function (FEV_1 ~50% predicted with SLT).
- 30% develop obliterative bronchiolitis within five years.

Bullectomy

There is still controversy over the indications for bullectomy and good results depend on careful patient selection. The ideal patient is young with a large bullae and minimal airway obstruction. In patients with COPD the problem is that surgical removal of one bulla leads to growth of other bullae as the emphysematous lung expands [42]. Favourable features are large bullae (>1 litre) with demonstration of surrounding lung compression and a lack of generalized emphysema demonstrated by computed tomography and a normal KCO.

Lung volume reduction surgery

Recently reduction of lung volume by excision has become popular for the treatment of severe emphysema. This involves resection of peripheral portions of both lungs using novel stapling techniques to prevent air leaks. The intention is to remove severely affected areas, thus allowing the remaining lung tissue to ventilate more effectively. This results in an increase in FEV_1 and a reduction in RV, with decreased dyspnoea, improved exercise tolerance and improved quality of life [43,44]. Careful patient selection is essential and patients with predominantly upper lobe involvement appear to do best. Although there is little information regarding long-term outcome of surgery, there is evidence that this treatment improves mortality and may be cost-effective [45]. A further benefit of this procedure is that it allows surgical resection in 'operable' lung cancers that would previously have been excluded because of poor lung function. Large randomized trials are currently underway.

References

1. American Thoracic Society. **Standards for the diagnosis and care of patients with chronic obstructive pulmonary disease.** *Am J Respir Crit Care Med* 1995; **152**:S77–S120.

2. Siafakis NM, Vermeire P, Pride NB *et al.* **Optimal assessment and management of chronic obstructive pulmonary disease (COPD).** *Eur Respir J* 1995; **8**:1398–1420.

3. British Thoracic Society. **BTS guidelines for the management of chronic obstructive pulmonary disease.** *Thorax* 1997; **52**(Suppl 5):S1–S28.

4. Pauwels RA, Buist AS, Calverley PMA *et al.* **Global strategy for the diagnosis, management and prevention of chronic obstructive pulmonary disease.** *Am J Respir Crit Care Med* 2001; **163**:1256–1276.

5. Scanlon PD, Connett JE, Waller LA *et al.* **Smoking cessation and lung function in mild-to-moderate chronic obstructive pulmonary disease. The Lung Health Study.** *Am J Respir Crit Care Med* 2000; **161**:381–390.

6. Lancaster T, Stead L, Silagy C *et al.* **Effectiveness of interventions to help people stop smoking: findings from the Cochrane Library.** *BMJ* 2000; **321**:355–358.

7. Silagy C, Mint D, Fowler G *et al.* **Beta-analysis on efficacy of nicotine replacement therapies in smoking cessation.** *Lancet* 1994; **343**:139–142.

8. West R, McNeill A, Raw M. **Smoking cessation guidelines for health professionals: an update. Health Education Authority.** *Thorax* 2000; **55**:987–999.

9. Jorenby DE, Leischow SJ, Nides MA *et al.* **A controlled trial of sustained-release bupropion, a nicotine patch, or both for smoking cessation.** *N Engl J Med* 1999; **340**:685–691.

10. Tashkin DP, Kanner R, Bailey W *et al.* **Smoking cessation in patients with chronic obstructive pulmonary disease: a double-blind, placebo-controlled, randomised trial.** *Lancet* 2001; **357**:1571–1575.

11. Holm KJ, Spencer CM. **Bupropion: a review of its use in the management of smoking cessation.** *Drugs* 2000; **59**:1007–1024.

12. Hughes JR, Stead LF, Lancaster T. **Antidepressants for smoking cessation (Cochrane Review).** *Cochrane Database Syst Rev* 2000; **4**:CD000031.

13. Anthonisen NR, Connett JE, Kiley JP *et al.* **Effects of smoking intervention and the use of an inhaled anticholinergic bronchodilator on the rate of decline of FEV_1.** *JAMA* 1994; **272**:1497–1505.

14. van Noord JA, de Munck DR, Bantje TA *et al.* **Long-term treatment of chronic obstructive pulmonary disease with salmeterol and the additive effect of ipratropium.** *Eur Respir J* 2000; **15**:878–885.

15. Chrystyn H, Mulley BA, Peake MD. **Dose response relation to oral theophylline in severe chronic obstructive airway disease.** *BMJ* 1988; **297**:1506–1510.

16. Anonymous. **In chronic obstructive pulmonary disease, a combination of ipratropium and salbutamol is more effective than either agent alone. An 85-day multicenter trial. COMBIVENT Inhalation Aerosol Study Group.** *Chest* 1994; **105**:1411–1419.

17. van der Palen J, Klein JJ, Kerkhoff AH *et al.* **Evaluation of the effectiveness of four different inhalers in patients with chronic obstructive pulmonary disease.** *Thorax* 1995; **50**:1183–1187.

18. Morrison JF, Jones PC, Muers MF. **Assessing physiological benefit from domiciliary nebulized bronchodilators in severe airflow limitation.** *Eur Respir J* 1992; **5**:424–429.

19. Wedzicha JA. **Effects of long-term oxygen therapy on neuropsychiatric function and quality of life.** *Respir Care* 2000; **45**:119–124.

20. Lock SH, Paul EA, Rudd RM *et al.* **Portable oxygen therapy: assessment and usage.** *Respir Med* 1991; **85**:407–412.

21. van Ede L, Yzermans CJ, Brouwer HJ. **Prevalence of depression in patients with chronic obstructive pulmonary disease: a systematic review.** *Thorax* 1999; **54**:688–692.

22. Smith K, Cook D, Guyatt GH *et al.* **Respiratory muscle training in chronic airflow limitation: a meta-analysis.** *Am Rev Respir Dis* 1992; **145**:533–539.

23. Clark CJ, Cochrane LM, Mackay E *et al.* **Skeletal muscle strength and endurance in patients with mild COPD and the effects of weight training.** *Eur Respir J* 2000; **15**:92–97.

24. Smith K, Cook D, Guyatt GH *et al.* **Respiratory muscle training in chronic airflow limitation: a meta-analysis.** *Am Rev Respir Dis* 1992; **145**:533–539.

25. Landbo C, Prescott E, Lange P *et al.* **Prognostic value of nutritional status in chronic obstructive pulmonary disease.** *Am J Respir Crit Care Med* 1999; **160**:1856–1861.

26. Ferreira IM, Brooks D, Lacasse Y *et al.* **Nutritional support for individuals with COPD: a meta-analysis.** *Chest* 2000; **117**:672–678.

27. Lacasse Y, Wong E, Guyatt GH *et al.* **Meta-analysis of respiratory rehabilitation in chronic obstructive pulmonary disease.** *Lancet* 1996; **348**:1115–1119.

28. Wedzicha JA, Bestall JC, Garrod R *et al.* **Randomized controlled trial of pulmonary rehabilitation in severe chronic obstructive pulmonary disease patients, stratified with the MRC dyspnoea scale.** *Eur Respir J* 1998; **12**:363–369.

29. Griffiths TL, Burr ML, Campbell IA *et al.* **Results at 1 year of outpatient multidisciplinary pulmonary rehabilitation: a randomised controlled trial.** *Lancet* 2000; **355**:362–368.

30. Bach PB, Brown C, Gelfand SE *et al.* **Management of acute exacerbations of chronic obstructive pulmonary disease: a summary and appraisal of published evidence.** *Ann Intern Med* 2001; **134**:600–620.

31. McCrory DC, Brown CD. **Inhaled short-acting beta2-agonists versus ipratropium for acute exacerbations of chronic obstructive pulmonary disease (Cochrane Review).** *Cochrane Database Syst Rev* 2001; **2**:CD002984.

32. Niewoehner DE, Erbland ML, Deupree RH *et al.* **Effect of systemic glucocorticoids on exacerbations of chronic obstructive pulmonary disease.** *N Engl J Med* 1999; **340**:1941–1947.

33. Davies L, Angus RM, Calverley PM. **Oral corticosteroids in patients admitted to hospital with exacerbations of chronic obstructive pulmonary disease: a prospective randomised controlled trial.** *Lancet* 1999; **354**:456–460.

34. Wood-Baker R, Walters EH, Gibson P. **Oral corticosteroids for acute exacerbations of chronic obstructive pulmonary disease (Cochrane Review).** *Cochrane Database Syst Rev* 2001; **2**:CD001288.

35. Jones SE, Packham S, Hebden M *et al.* **Domiciliary nocturnal intermittent positive pressure ventilation in patients with respiratory failure due to severe COPD: long-term follow up and effect on survival.** *Thorax* 1998; **53**:495–498.

36. Doherty MJ, Greenstone MA. **Survey of non-invasive ventilation (NIPPV) in patients with acute exacerbations of chronic obstructive pulmonary disease (COPD) in the UK.** *Thorax* 1998; **53**:863–866.

37. Bott J, Carroll ND, Conway JH *et al.* **Randomised controlled trial of nasal ventilation in acute ventilatory failure due to chronic obstructive airways disease.** *Lancet* 1993; **341**:1555–1557.

38. Brochard L, Mancebo J, Wysocki M *et al.* **Noninvasive ventilation for acute exacerbations of chronic obstructive pulmonary disease.** *N Engl J Med* 1995; **333**:817–822.

39. Edelman JD, Kotloff RM. **Surgical approaches to advanced emphysema.** *Respir Care Clin N Am* 1998; **4**:513–539.

40. Trulock EP. **Lung transplantation for COPD.** *Chest* 1998; **113**:269S–276S.

41. Maurer JR, Frost AE, Estenne M *et al.* **International guidelines for the selection of lung transplant candidates. The International Society for Heart and Lung Transplantation, the American Thoracic Society, the American Society of Transplant Physicians, the European Respiratory Society.** *Heart Lung* 1998; **27**:223–229.

42. Mehran RJ, Deslauriers J. **Indications for surgery and patient work-up for bullectomy.** *Chest Surg Clin N Am* 1995; **5**:717–734.

43. Doyle RL, Mark JB. **Lung volume reduction surgery for the treatment of chronic obstructive pulmonary disease.** *Adv Intern Med* 1998; **43**:233–252.

44. Geddes D, Davies M, Koyama H *et al.* **Effect of lung-volume-reduction surgery in patients with severe emphysema.** *N Engl J Med* 2000; **343**:239–245.

45. Meyers BF, Yusen RD, Lefrak SS *et al.* **Improved long-term survival seen after lung volume reduction surgery compared to continued medical therapy for emphysema.** *Ann Thorac Surg* 2001; **71**:2081.

Chapter 5

Future trends in therapy

There have been relatively few advances in the therapeutic options for the treatment of COPD, but better understanding of the molecular mechanisms involved in the pathogenesis of COPD will undoubtedly lead to improved therapies in the future [1,2].

New bronchodilators

Bronchodilators are the mainstay of current management of COPD and the major recent advances have been in the development of long-acting bronchodilators.

New anticholinergics

The existence of several subtypes of muscarinic receptors in airways has suggested that more selective muscarinic antagonists may have advantages over the existing non-selective drugs, such as ipratropium bromide and oxitropium bromide [3] (*see* Figure 5.1). First, M_1-receptors are localized to parasympathetic ganglia and their blockade results in reduced reflex bronchoconstriction. Second, M_2-receptors located at cholinergic nerve terminals inhibit the release of acetylcholine, thus acting as autoreceptors (*see* Figure 5.2). Third, M_3-receptors mediate the bronchoconstrictor and mucus secretion action of acetylcholine in human airways.

Non-selective anticholinergic drugs, such as atropine and ipratropium bromide, block M_1- and M_3-receptors, leading to bronchodilatation. However, by blocking pre-junctional M_2-receptors this leads to an increase in acetylcholine release and this may work against the post-junctional blockade of M_3-receptors, making these antagonists less efficient. It has been difficult to develop M_3-selective antagonists. Darifencin (UK-88525) is M_3-selective and is in clinical development [4]. Revatropate (UK-112166) is an M_1/M_3 antagonist in clinical development as a bronchodilator for COPD [4]. However, neither drug is very selective and both have a short duration of action and are apparently not being further developed.

Tiotropium bromide

The most interesting bronchodilator in development is tiotropium bromide, which has the unique property of kinetic selectivity, with rapid dissociation from M_2-receptors and very slow dissociation from M_1- and M_3-receptors [5–7]. Tiotropium bromide is a quaternary ammonium derivative like ipratropium bromide (*see* Figure 5.3). The most interesting property of tiotropium bromide is its very long duration of action. It has a high affinity and dissociates very slowly from M_1- and M_3-receptors in human lung and produces long-term blockade of cholinergic neural bronchoconstriction in human airway smooth muscle. However, its effects on acetylcholine release are short-lived, confirming functional selectivity for M_3- compared with M_2-receptors. In studies of patients with COPD, single doses of tiotropium bromide give prolonged bronchodilatation, lasting over 24 hours [8] (*see* Figure 5.4).

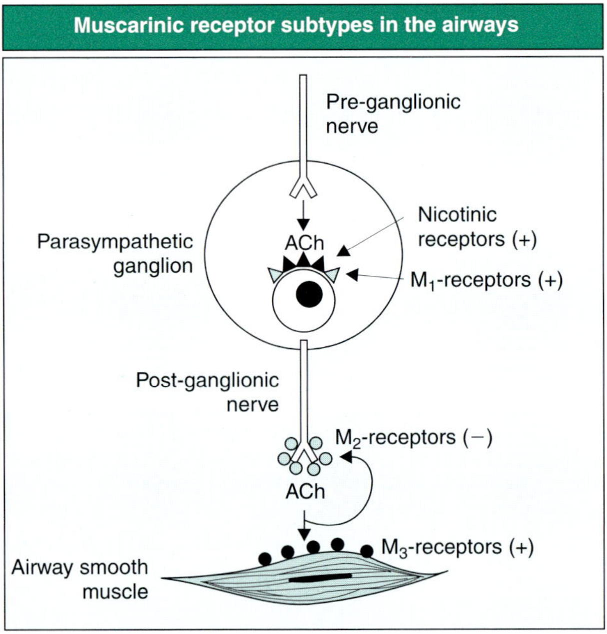

Figure 5.1. M_1 receptors are localized in parasympathetic ganglia and augment ganglionic transmission, M_2 receptors are at cholinergic nerve terminals an inhibit acetylcholine (ACh) release, whereas M_3 receptors are in muscle (and mucus glands) and mediate bronchoconstriction (and mucus secretion).

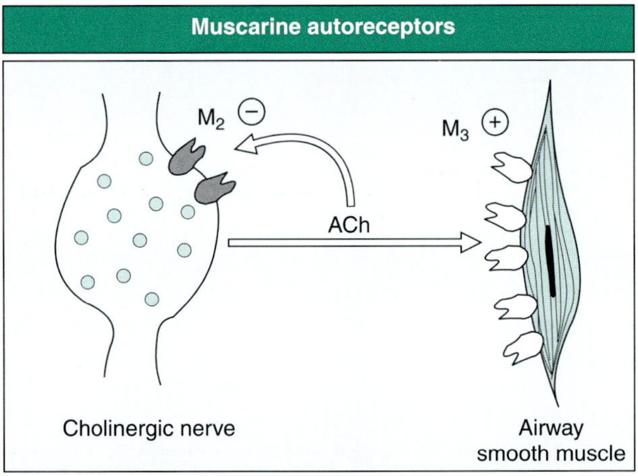

Figure 5.2. Acetylcholine released from cholinergic nerves causes bronchoconstriction via M_3 receptors, but also acts on M_2 receptors on the nerve to inhibit release. A non-selective anticholinergic, such as atropine or ipratropium bromide, blocks both M_2 and M_3 receptors and therefore may be less effective that a selective M_3 receptor antagonist.

Figure 5.3. Bronchodilator effect of a single dose of tiotropium bromide in patients with chronic obstructive pulmonary disease (COPD). Adapted from [8].

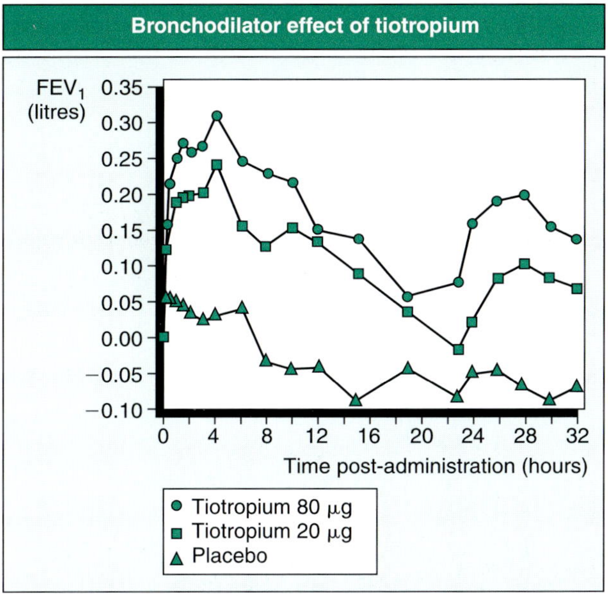

Figure 5.4. Once daily administration of tiotropium bromide (18 μg; n=180) is more effective than four times daily administration of ipratropium bromide (40 μg; n=91) in patients with chronic obstructive pulmonary disease (COPD). PEF, peak expiratory flow. Adapted from [11].

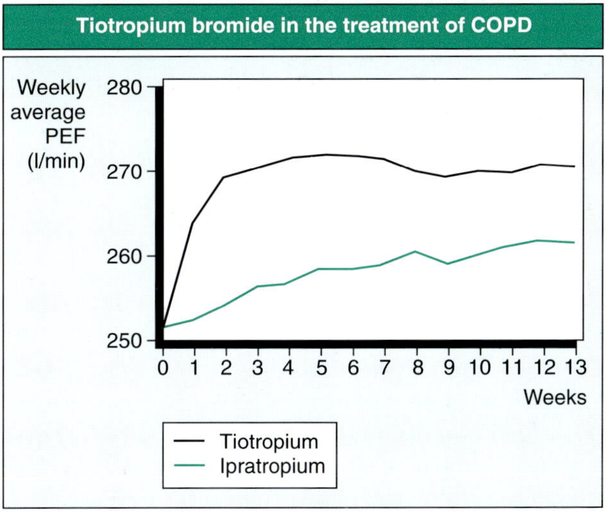

Clinical studies have shown that tiotropium bromide given as a once daily inhalation is effective in improving lung function and symptoms of patients with COPD and is more effective than β_2-agonists and ipratropium bromide given four times daily [9–11] (*see* Figure 5.5). This demonstrates that tiotropium bromide will be suitable for once daily dosing and that it will soon be available as a once daily dry powder

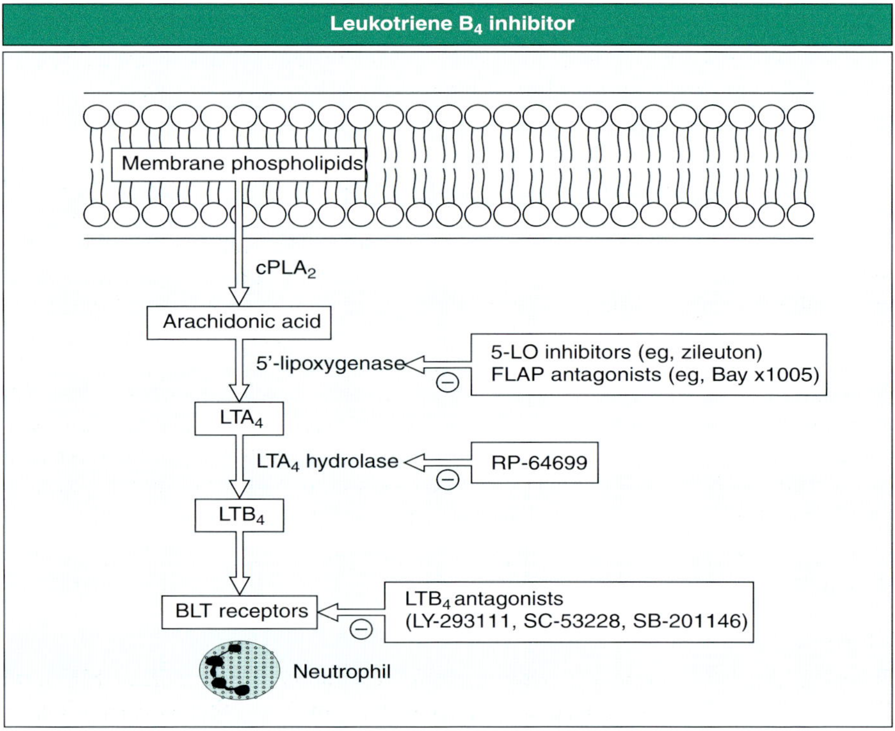

Figure 5.5. Drugs that block leukotriene B_4 (LTB_4) receptors (BLT), and LTB_4 generation should be effective. 5-LO, 5'-lipoxygenase.

inhalation [7]. It is likely to become the bronchodilator of choice for COPD in the future. Side effects are not a problem as the drug is not absorbed and the incidence of dry mouth is similar to that seen with ipratropium bromide [11].

Long-acting β_2-agonists

Long-acting inhaled β_2-agonists salmeterol and formoterol are beneficial in patients with COPD, with improved lung function and symptom control, as discussed in Chapter 2. There is now a search for a once-daily inhaled β_2-agonist. Bambuterol, an oral once-daily β_2-agonist, may also be useful.

Viozan

AR-C68397AA (Viozan), a dual agonist of β_2-adrenergic and dopamine D_2 receptors, has been in clinical development for the treatment of COPD [12]. The rationale for the development of Viozan is that D_2-agonists may activate receptors on airway sensory nerves to inhibit cough and reflex mucus secretion. Clinical studies have not demonstrated clinical benefit over β_2-agonists alone [13].

Mediator antagonists

Several mediators are involved in the pathophysiology of COPD, and antagonists to individual mediators have now been developed or are in development.

LTB_4 inhibitors

LTB_4 is a potent chemoattractant of neutrophils and is increased in the sputum of patients with COPD [14]. It may be inhibited in several ways (*see* Figure 5.5). Selective LTB_4 receptor (BLT receptor) antagonists have now been developed. A potent LTB_4 antagonist (LY-293111) is ineffective against allergen challenge in patients with asthma, although it inhibits the neutrophil recruitment into the airways during the late response, indicating the capacity to inhibit neutrophil chemotaxis in the airways [15]. Several potent LTB_4 antagonists are now in development (including SC-53228, CP-105696, SB-201146, BIIL284). LTB_4 is synthesized by 5′-lipoxygenase (5-LO), of which there are now several potent inhibitors. 5-LO inhibitors, such as zileuton, are now available in some countries for the treatment of asthma, since they also inhibit the synthesis of cysteinyl-leukotrienes, but it is not certain whether they are effective in COPD. Several selective 5-LO inhibitors are in clinical development.

LTA_4 hydrolase inhibitors that selectively inhibit the synthesis of LTB_4 have been developed.

Chemokine inhibitors

Several chemokines are involved in neutrophil chemotaxis [16,17]. These belong to the CXC family of chemokines and the most prominent member is IL-8, which is markedly elevated in the sputum of patients with COPD [18]. IL-8 activates a low affinity specific receptor (CXCR1) and more potently a receptor that is activated by other CXC chemokines. A potent non-peptide inhibitor of IL-8 has been developed [19,20]. Other CXC chemokines, such as GRO-α, are also elevated in COPD and therefore a CXCR2 antagonist is likely to be more useful than a CXCRI antagonist, particularly as CXCR2 are also expressed on monocytes. Small molecule inhibitors of CXCR2, such as SB-225002, have now been developed [19,20].

TNF-α inhibitors

TNF-α levels are raised in the sputum of COPD patients [21]. The severe wasting that occurs in some patients with advanced COPD might be due to skeletal muscle apoptosis, resulting from increased circulating TNF-α. Patients with COPD and cachexia have increased release of TNF-α from circulating leukocytes [22]. Humanized monoclonal TNF antibodies (infliximab) and soluble TNF receptors (etanercept) that are effective in other chronic inflammatory diseases, such as rheumatoid arthritis and inflammatory bowel disease, should also be effective in COPD [23,24]. There may be problems with long-term administration because of the development of blocking antibodies. Repeated injections are also inconvenient. TNF-α converting enzyme (TACE), which is required for the release of soluble TNF-α, may be a more attractive target because it is possible to discover small molecule TACE inhibitors, some of which are also matrix metalloproteinase

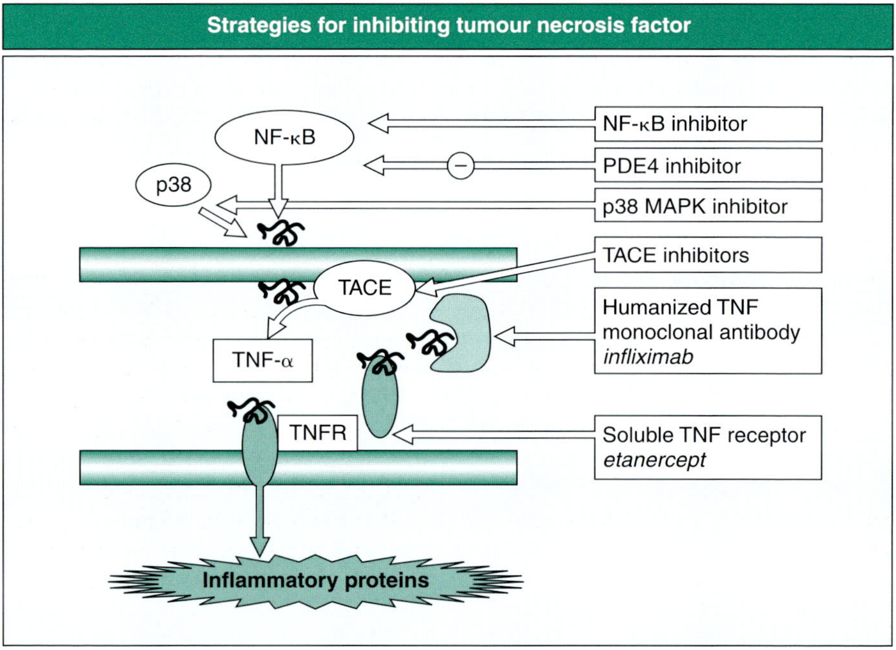

Figure 5.6. TNF, tumour necrosis factor; NFκB, nuclear factor-κB; TACE, tumour necrosis factor-alpha converting enzyme; PDE, phosphodiesterase; TNFR, tumour necrosis factor receptor.

inhibitors [25] (*see* Figure 5.6). General anti-inflammatory drugs such as phosphodiesterase inhibitors and p38 inhibitors also potently inhibit TNF-α expression.

Antioxidants

As oxidative stress is important in COPD, particularly during exacerbations, antioxidants may be of use in the therapy of COPD. N-acetyl cysteine provides cysteine for enhanced production of glutathione (GSH) and has antioxidant effects *in vitro* and *in vivo*. Antioxidants that are more effective, including stable glutathione compounds and selenium-based drugs, are now in development for clinical use [26].

Inducible nitric oxide synthase inhibitors

Oxidative stress and increased nitric oxide release from expression of inducible nitric oxide synthase (iNOS) may result in the formation of peroxynitrite, which is a potent radical and may nitrate proteins, resulting in altered function. 3-Nitrotyrosine may indicate peroxynitrite formation and is markedly increased in sputum macrophages of patients with COPD [27]. Selective inhibitors of iNOS are now in development [28].

Anti-inflammatory treatments

COPD is characterized by inflammation of the airways, with activated T lymphocytes, and increased numbers of macrophages and neutrophils. Corticosteroids are largely ineffective (*see* Chapter 3), prompting the search for new anti-inflammatory drugs. There are several approaches to inhibiting inflammation (*see* Table 5.1 and Figure 5.7).

Phosphodiesterase inhibitors

Phosphodiesterases (PDEs) break down cyclic nucleotides (cyclic AMP and cyclic GMP) that regulate cellular activity. Inhibition of these enzymes results in inhibition of inflammatory cells and relaxation of smooth muscle. Over nine families of PDEs are now recognised, but the family most relevant to COPD inflammation is PDE4, because PDE4 inhibitors inhibit neutrophilic inflammation, and also inhibit the function of macrophages and T lymphocytes [29]. PDE4 inhibitors also have a bronchodilator action (*see* Figure 5.8). Preliminary studies suggest that a selective PDE4 inhibitor, cilomilast, has some beneficial clinical effect in patients with COPD and larger studies are currently underway [30]. PDE4 inhibitors are limited by side effects, particularly nausea and other gastrointestinal effects, but it might be possible to develop isoenzyme subtype selective inhibitors in the future, which are less likely to be dose limited by adverse effects.

NF-κB inhibitors

The transcription factor NF-κB regulates the expression of IL-8 and other chemokines, TNF-α, and some matrix metalloproteinases. There are several possible approaches to inhibition of NF-κB. Research in this field has focused on gene transfer of the inhibitor of NF-κB (IκB); a search for inhibitors of IκB kinases, NF-κB-inducing kinase and IκB

Inhibitors of inflammation
LTB_4 antagonists (LY-29311, SC-53228, CP-105696, SB-201146)
Interleukin-8 inhibitors (interleukin-8 synthesis inhibitors, CXC receptor antagonists)
TNF-inhibitors (monoclonal antibodies, soluble receptors, TNF convertase inhibitors)
Antioxidants (N-acetyl cysteine, glutathione analogues, vitamins C and E, nitrones)
Phosphodiesterase-4 inhibitors (ciclesonide, CP-80633, CDP-840)
NF-κB inhibitors (IκB kinase inhibitors, IκB-α gene transfer)
Adhesion molecule inhibitors (anti CD11/CD18, anti-ICAM-1, E-selectin inhibitors)
Interleukin-10
p38 MAP kinase inhibitors
Phosphoinositide-3 kinase-γ inhibitors

Table 5.1. LTB_4, leukotriene B_4; TNF, tumour necrosis factor; NF-κB, nuclear factor-κB; IκB, inhibitor of nuclear factor-κB.

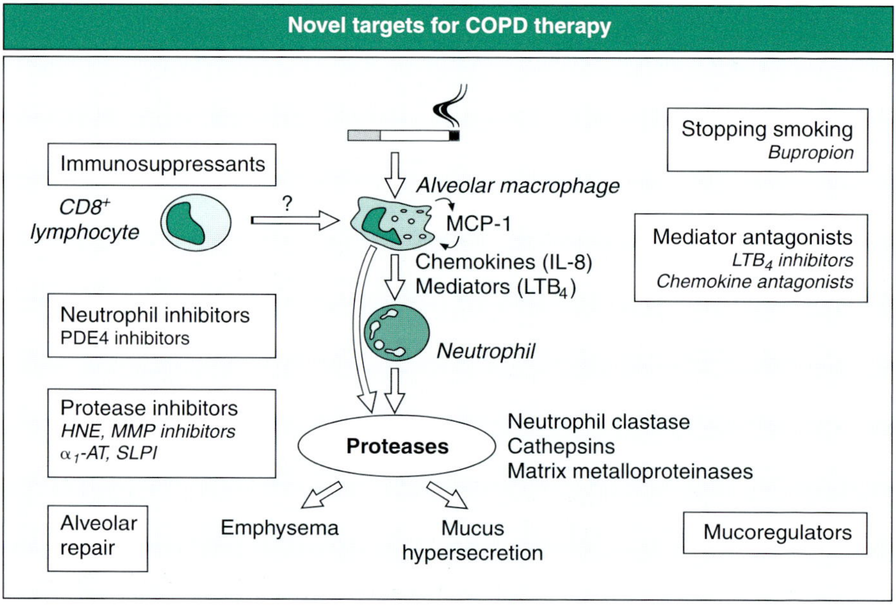

Figure 5.7. IL, interleukin; PDE, phosphodiesterase; LT, leukotriene, HNE, human neutrophil elastase; MMP, matrix metalloproteinase; α_1-AT, alpha-1-antitrypsin, SLPI, secretory leukoprotease inhibitor.

ubiquitin ligase, which regulate the activity of NF-κB; and the development of drugs that inhibit the degradation of IκB [31]. One concern about this approach is that effective inhibitors of NF-κB may result in immune suppression and impair host defences, because knock-out mice that lack NF-κB succumb to septicaemia. However, there are alternative pathways of NF-κB activation that might be more important in inflammatory disease [32].

Adhesion molecule blockers

Recruitment of neutrophils, monocytes and cytotoxic T cells into the lungs and respiratory tract is dependent on adhesion molecules expressed on these cells and on endothelial cells in the pulmonary and bronchial circulations. Several adhesion molecules can now be inhibited pharmacologically. For example, E-selectin on endothelial cells interacts with sialyl-Lewis^x on neutrophils. A mimic of sialyl-Lewis^x, TBC 1269, blocks selectins and inhibits granulocyte adhesion, with preferential effects on neutrophils [33]. However, there are concerns about this therapeutic approach for a chronic disease, as an impaired neutrophilic response may increase the patient's susceptibility to infections. The expression of Mac-1 (CD11b/CD18) is increased on neutrophils of patients with COPD, suggesting that targeting this adhesion molecule, which is also expressed on monocytes and macrophages, might be beneficial [34].

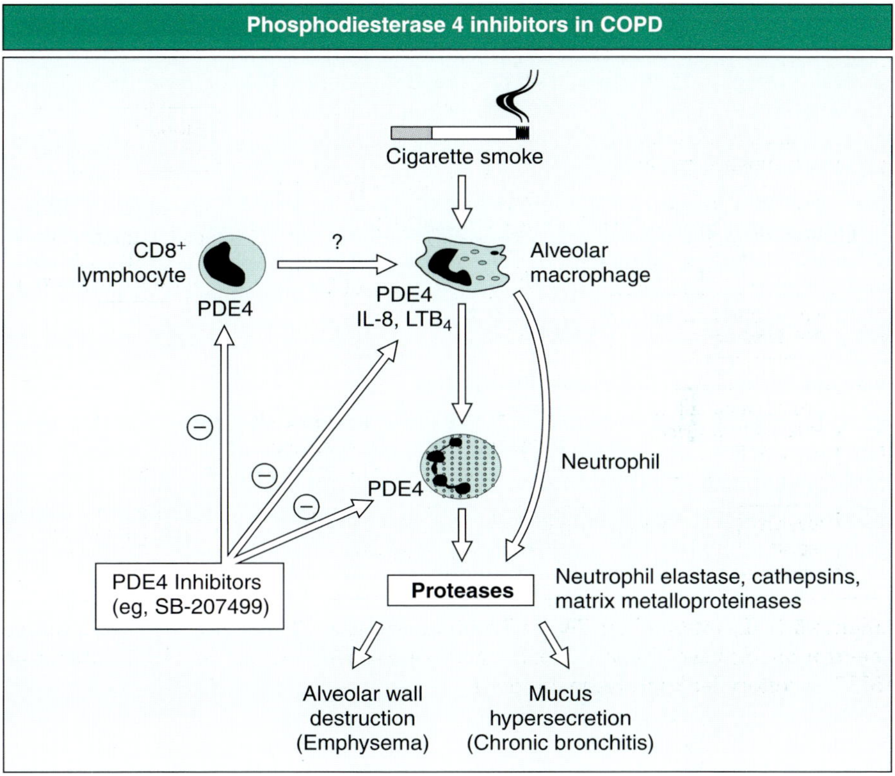

Figure 5.8. Phosphodiesterase-4 (PDE4) inhibitors may have several beneficial effects, acting on neutrophils, macrophages and $CD8^+$ lymphocytes.

Interleukin-10

IL-10 is a cytokine with a wide range of anti-inflammatory actions. It inhibits the secretion of TNF-α and IL-8 from macrophages, but tips the balance in favour of antiproteases, by decreasing the expression of matrix metalloproteinases, while increasing the expression of endogenous tissue inhibitors of matrix metalloproteinases (TIMPs). IL-10 concentrations are reduced in induced sputum from patients with COPD; this may therefore be a mechanism for increasing lung inflammation [35]. IL-10 is currently in clinical trials for other chronic inflammatory diseases (eg, inflammatory bowel disease, rheumatoid arthritis and psoriasis), including patients with steroid resistance, but IL-10 may cause haematological side effects [36]. Treatment with daily injections of IL-10 over several weeks has been well tolerated. IL-10 may have therapeutic potential in COPD, especially if a selective activator of IL-10 receptors or signal transduction pathways can be developed.

p38 mitogen-activated protein kinase inhibitors

Mitogen-activated protein (MAP) kinases play a key role in chronic inflammation and several complex enzyme cascades have now been defined. One of these, the p38 MAP kinase pathway, is involved in the expression of inflammatory cytokines, including IL-8, TNF-α and MMPs [37,38]. Non-peptide inhibitors of p38 MAP kinase, such as SB-203580, SB-239063 and RWJ-67657, have now been developed and these drugs have a broad range of anti-inflammatory effects [39]. SB-239063 reduces neutrophil infiltration after inhaled endotoxin and concentrations of IL-6 and MMP-9 in broncho-alveolar lavage fluid of rats, indicating its potential as an anti-inflammatory agent in COPD [40]. It is likely that such a broad-spectrum anti-inflammatory drug will have some toxicity, but inhalation may be a feasible therapeutic approach.

Phosphoinositide 3-kinase inhibitors

Phosphoinositide 3-kinase inhibitors (PI-3Ks) are a family of enzymes that lead to the generation of lipid second messengers that regulate a number of cellular events. A particular isoform, PI-3Kγ, is involved in neutrophil recruitment and activation. Knock-out of the PI-3Kγ gene results in inhibition of neutrophil migration and activation, as well as impaired T lymphocyte and macrophage function [41]. This suggests that selective PI-3Kγ inhibitors may have relevant anti-inflammatory activity in COPD.

Protease inhibitors

There is compelling evidence for an imbalance between proteases that digest elastin (and other structural proteins) and antiproteases that protect against this in COPD. This suggests that either inhibiting these proteolytic enzymes or increasing antiproteases may be beneficial and theoretically should prevent the progression of airflow obstruction in COPD. Considerable progress has been made in identifying the enzymes involved in elastolytic activity in emphysema and in characterizing the endogenous antiproteases that counteract this activity [42,43] (*see* Table 5.2.).

Enzyme inhibitors for COPD therapy
Enzyme inhibitors
Neutrophil elastase inhibitors (ICI-200355, ONO-5046)
Cathepsin inhibitors (suramin)
MMP inhibitors (batimastat, marimastat, selective MMP inhibitors)
Endogenous antiproteases
α_1-Antitrypsin (purified, human recombinant, gene transfer)
Elafin
Secretory leukoprotease inhibitor (human recombinant)

Table 5.2. COPD, chronic obstructive pulmonary disease; MMP, matrix metalloproteinase.

Neutrophil elastase inhibitors

As neutrophil elastase is a major constituent of lung elastolytic activity and also potently stimulates mucus secretion, it is a potential target for inhibition. Several potent neutrophil elastase inhibitors have been developed, including peptide inhibitors, such as ICI-200355, and non-peptide inhibitors, such as ONO-5046. There are few clinical studies in COPD; the neutrophil elastase inhibitor MR889 administered for four weeks showed no overall effect on plasma elastin-derived peptides or urinary desmosine (markers of elastolytic activity) [44]. It may be difficult to inhibit enzyme activity as neutrophils adhere to connective tissue, so that access of the enzyme inhibitor may be a problem. Intracellular inhibitors may be more effective.

Although neutrophil elastase is likely to be the major mechanism mediating elastolysis in patients with alpha-1-antitrypsin (α_1-AT) deficiency, it may well not be the major elastolytic enzyme in smoking-related COPD, and it is important to consider other enzymes, such as cathepsins and proteinase-3, as targets for inhibition.

Matrix metalloproteinase inhibitors

Matrix metalloproteinases (MMPs) derived from macrophages, neutrophils and epithelial cells may also play a role in connective tissue destruction, suggesting that MMP inhibitors may be beneficial. There are several approaches to inhibiting MMPs [45]. One approach is to enhance the secretion of the endogenous inhibitors of MMPs — TIMPs. Another is to develop enzyme inhibitors, such as batimastat (BB-94) and the orally active marimastat (BB-2516). These are non-selective inhibitors and have side effects. Selective inhibitors of individual MMPs, such as MMP-9 and MMP-12 (metalloelastase), are now in development and are likely to be better tolerated in therapy for patients with chronic disease.

α_1-Antitrypsin

The association of α_1-AT deficiency with early-onset emphysema suggested that this endogenous inhibitor of neutrophil elastase may be of therapeutic benefit in COPD. Cigarette smoking may inactivate α_1-AT, resulting in unopposed activity of neutrophil elastase and cathepsins. Extraction of α_1-AT from human plasma is very expensive and extracted α_1-antitrypsin is only available in a few countries. This treatment has to be given intravenously and has a half-life of only five days. Human α_1-AT has now been available for over 10 years, but even in patients with severe α_1-AT deficiency and emphysema, there is only a marginal effect on the rate of decline in FEV_1 [46]. Inhaled α_1-AT formulations, although these are inefficient and expensive [47]. Recombinant α_1-AT with amino acid substitutions to increase stability may result in a more stable product. Gene therapy is another possibility using an adenovirus vector or liposomes, but there have been major problems in developing efficient delivery systems. There is a particular problem with gene transfer in α_1-AT deficiency in that large amounts of protein (1–2 g) need to be synthesized each day. There is no evidence that α_1-AT treatment would halt the progression of COPD and emphysema in patients who have normal plasma concentrations.

Serpins

Other serum protease inhibitors (serpins), such as elafin, may also be important in counteracting elastolytic activity in the lung. Elafin, an elastase-specific inhibitor is found in bronchoalveolar lavage and is synthesized by epithelial cells in response to inflammatory stimuli [48]. Serpins may not be able to inhibit neutrophil elastase at the sites of elastin destruction, due to tight adherence of the inflammatory cell to connective tissue. Furthermore, these proteins may become inactivated by the inflammatory process and the action of oxidants, so that they may not be able to counteract elastolytic activity in the lung unless used in conjunction with other therapies.

Secretory leukoprotease inhibitor

Secretory leukoprotease inhibitor (SLPI) is a 12 kDa serpin that appears to be a major inhibitor of elastase activity in the airways. It is secreted by epithelial cells [48]. In-vitro recombinant human SLPI is more effective at inhibiting neutrophil mediated proteolysis than α_1-AT [49]. Recombinant human SLPI given by aerosolization increases anti-neutrophil elastase activity in epithelial lining fluid for over 12 hours, indicating potential therapeutic use [50].

Mucoregulators

Increased secretion of mucus is found in all patients who smoke heavily, irrespective of airflow obstruction. However, recent epidemiological data suggests that mucus hypersecretion is significantly associated with a more rapid decline in FEV_1 and increased hospitalization of patients with COPD [51]. This suggests that it may be important to develop drugs that inhibit the hypersecretion of mucus, although it is important to find drugs that do not suppress the normal mucus secretion or impair mucociliary clearance. There are several types of mucoregulatory drug in development.

Tachykinin antagonists

Tachykinins are potent stimulants of mucus secretion from submucosal glands and goblet cells in human and animal airways and act via neurokinin $(NK)_1$-receptors. In animal studies cigarette smoke induces airway mucus secretion via release of tachykinins from sensory nerves through a local axon reflex mechanism [52]. NK_1-antagonists markedly inhibit neurogenic mucus secretion and may therefore have potential as mucoregulators in cigarette smoke-induced chronic bronchitis. Several potent non-peptide NK_1-receptor antagonists, such as CP-99994 and SR-140333, are now in clinical development, and might have a role as regulators of mucus hypersecretion in COPD.

Sensory neuropeptide release inhibitors

Another approach to blocking tachykinin-mediated effects is to inhibit the release of tachykinins from sensory nerve endings, via activation of pre-junctional receptors [53]. Of these receptors, μ-opioid receptors are most effective and the μ-opioid agonist morphine potently inhibits cigarette smoke-induced mucus secretion in animal airways. In human airways *in vitro* morphine inhibits mucus secretion activated via stimulation of sensory nerves [54]. Although morphine itself may not be useful as a therapeutic agent because of addiction, peripherally acting opioid agonists that do not cross the blood–brain barrier, such as BW443, might be of use. Many pre-junctional receptors appear to operate via the opening of a common potassium (K^+) channel, suggesting that K^+ channel openers may be useful in blocking mucus secretion. Openers of ATP-dependent K^+ channels, such as levcromakalim, have an inhibitory effect on cigarette smoke-induced mucus secretion in animals [55].

Mediator and enzyme inhibitors

Many mediators stimulate mucus secretion from submucosal glands and/or goblet cells and may therefore contribute to increased mucus secretion in COPD. It is unlikely, however, that any mediator antagonists (eg, anti-leukotrienes) would have a major effect on mucus secretion. Neutrophil elastase, proteinase-3 and other proteases are potent stimulants of submucosal gland and goblet cell secretion, suggesting that protease inhibitors may have inhibitory effects on mucus secretion, as well as inhibiting lung destruction. Inhalation of the COX inhibitor indomethacin is reported to reduce mucus hypersecretion in patients with COPD [56], but long-term trials of COX inhibitors have not yet been undertaken.

MUC gene suppressors

Nine MUC genes that code for mucin synthesis have already been cloned and many are expressed in human airways [57]. MUC5AC (particularly in goblet cells), MUC5B (particularly in submucosal glands), MUC4 and MUC8 appear to be important in airway mucus. MUC5AC may be up-regulated by inflammatory cytokines and inhibited by glucocorticoids [58]. It is possible that drugs may be developed that inhibit the abnormally increased expression of MUC genes in COPD, while preserving baseline secretion of MUC2. Such drugs, other than corticosteroids, have not yet been developed.

Macrolide antibiotics

Erythromycin inhibits mucin secretion from human airways *in vitro* and appears to be interactive with corticosteroids [59]. This property does not appear to be related to their antibiotic activity and is consistent with other studies demonstrating an inhibitory action of erythromycin on cell secretion. The molecular mechanisms involved in these effects need to be defined, and controlled studies in COPD may be indicated.

Epidermal growth factors antagonists

EGF appears to play an important role in mucus secretion and increased expression of MUC genes [60,61]. This suggests that inhibition of EGF receptors or signalling pathways may be effective treatments for mucus hypersecretion.

Drug delivery

Bronchodilators are currently administered using inhalers, MDIs or DPIs that have been optimized to deliver drugs to the respiratory tract in asthma. In emphysema, however, the inflammatory and destructive process takes place in the lung parenchyma. This implies that if a drug is to be delivered by inhalation then it should have a lower mass median diameter, so that there is preferential deposition in the lung periphery. It may be more appropriate to give therapy parenterally since it will need to reach the lung parenchyma via the pulmonary circulation, but parenteral administration may increase the risk of systemic side effects.

In the future targeted delivery may be more effective with a reduced risk of side effects. For example, drugs may be delivered that are selectively taken up by macrophages, which play such a critical role in the pathogenesis of COPD. This would reduce the risk of side effects, which may be quite high for drugs such as NF-κB and p38 MAP kinase inhibitors.

New technologies

Artificial ventilation devices have improved enormously. Non-invasive ventilation using NIPPV has been an important advance in the management of acute exacerbations of COPD in hospital, and more recently in the control of hypercapnic respiratory failure at home, thus reducing the need for hospitalization [62]. NIPPV corrects the hypercapnia and respiratory acidosis, while resting the respiratory muscles. Excellent results in management of acute exacerbations have been reported, with significant reduction in mortality and time spent in hospital.

Early detection

One of the most important developments in the future will be the detection of COPD at an earlier stage before symptoms appear. This will depend on screening of cigarette smokers in the community and instituting preventive measure (smoking cessation plans and possible drug therapy). More rigorous attempts to prevent smoking (particularly in teenagers) with a complete ban on cigarette advertising and increased taxation of tobacco, are needed. In the future it may be possible to detect the genetic polymorphisms that predetermine whether a patient will develop COPD with cigarette smoking. The development of small lungs in neonates, due to malnutrition and maternal smoking in pregnancy, may increase the risk of COPD in cigarette smoking and emphasizes the importance of trying to prevent cigarette smoking by pregnant women.

Future directions

New drugs for the treatment of COPD are needed. Although preventing and quitting smoking is the obvious preferred approach, this has proved to be very difficult for the majority of patients and even with the use of bupropion only approximately 15% of patients become sustained quitters [63]. In addition, it is likely that the inflammatory process initiated by cigarette smoking may continue even when smoking has ceased [64]. Furthermore, COPD may be due to other environmental factors (eg, cooking fumes, pollutants, passive smoking, other inhaled toxins) or due to developmental changes in the lungs.

Genetic risk factors

It is likely that several genetic polymorphisms will discovered that will confer risk on smokers for the development of COPD and emphysema. Eventually it will eventually be possible to identify at risk patients and to focus more effective therapies on these patients before lung function becomes seriously impaired. The development of gene chip technologies that allow the detection of multiple polymorphisms may provide a simple way to detect the risk in individual patients. It may also predict the risk of developing pulmonary hypertension and cor pulmonale.

Drugs affecting remodelling

Since a major mechanism of airway obstruction in COPD is loss of elastic recoil due to proteolytic destruction of lung parenchyma, it seems unlikely that this could be reversible by drug therapy, although it might be possible to reduce the rate of progression by preventing the inflammatory and enzymatic disease process. Retinoic acid increases the number of alveoli in rats and, remarkably, reverses the histological and physiological changes induced by elastase treatment [65]. It is not certain whether such alveolar proliferation is possible in adult human lungs, however. Inhalation of retinoic acid or its derivatives may be preferred because side effects are likely to be problem with repeated administrations [66]. Retinoic acid activates intracellular retinoic acid receptors, which act as transcription factors to regulate the expression of many genes. A particular subtype of retinoic acid receptor appears to mediate this effect, and selective agonists, which would be safer than all-trans retinoic acid, are in development [67]. The molecular mechanisms involved and whether this can be extrapolated to humans is not yet known. Several retinoic acid receptor subtype agonists have now been developed that may have a greater selectivity for this effect. Hepatic growth factor (scatter factor) appears to be a major growth factor responsible for alveolar development, and alveolar cells respond to it during lung development [68]. If responsiveness could be restored, this might be a strategy for repairing damaged lungs.

Monitoring the effects of therapy

Several drugs are now in development may be useful in COPD. These include LTB_4 antagonists and 5-lipoxygenase inhibitors, PDE4 inhibitors, new antioxidants and neutrophil elastase and MMP inhibitors. It will be difficult to demonstrate the efficacy of such treatments as determination of the effect of any drug on the rate of decline in lung function will require large studies over at least two years. There is an urgent need to develop surrogate markers, such as analysis of sputum parameters (cells, mediators, enzymes), that may predict the clinical usefulness of such drugs. Non-invasive markers of inflammation in COPD, including volatile gases and breath condensate, are also in development [69].

References

1. Barnes PJ. **Novel approaches and targets for treatment of chronic obstructive pulmonary disease.** *Am J Respir Crit Care Med* 1999; **160**:S72–S79.

2. Barnes PJ. **New treatments for COPD.** *Curr Opin Pharmacol* 2001; **1**:217–222.

3. Barnes PJ. **Muscarinic receptor subtypes in airways.** *Life Sci* 1993; **52**:521–528.

4. Alabaster VA. **Discovery and development of selective M_3 antagonists for clinical use.** *Life Sci* 1997; **60**:1053–1060.

5. Disse B, Speck GA, Rominger KL *et al.* **Tiotropium (Spiriva): mechanistical considerations and clinical profile in obstructive lung disease.** *Life Sci* 1999; **64**:457–464.

6. Barnes PJ. **The pharmacological properties of tiotropium.** *Chest* 2000; **117**:63S–66S.

7. Barnes PJ. **Tiotropium bromide.** *Expert Opin Investig Drugs* 2001; **10**:733–740.

8. Maesen FPV, Smeets JJ, Sledsens TJM *et al.* **Tiotropium bromide, a new long-acting antimuscarinic bronchodilator: a pharmacodynamic study in patients with chronic obstructive pulmonary disease (COPD).** *Eur Respir J* 1995; **8**:1506–1513.

9. Littner MR, Ilowite JS, Tashkin DP *et al.* **Long-acting bronchodilation with once-daily dosing of tiotropium (Spiriva) in stable chronic obstructive pulmonary disease.** *Am J Respir Crit Care Med* 2000; **161**:1136–1142.

10. Casaburi R, Briggs DDJ, Donohue JF *et al.* **The spirometric efficacy of once-daily dosing with tiotropium in stable COPD : a 13-week multicenter trial.** *Chest* 2000; **118**:1294–1302.

11. van Noord JA, Bantje TA, Eland ME *et al.* **A randomised controlled comparison of tiotropium and ipratropium in the treatment of chronic obstructive pulmonary disease. The Dutch Tiotropium Study Group.** *Thorax* 2000; **55**:289–294.

12. Newbold P, Jackson DM, Young A *et al.* **Dual D2 dopamine receptor and β_2-adrenceptor agonists for the modulation of sensory nerves in COPD.** In: *New Drugs for Asthma and COPD.* Edited by TT Hansel and PJ Barnes. Basel: Karger, 2001;68–71.

13. Hasani A, Toms N, Agnew JE *et al.* **The effect of multiple doses of Viozan (AR-C68397AA) compared with salbutamol on lung mucociliary clearance and sputum production in patients with COPD [Abstract].** *Am J Respir Crit Care Med* 2000; **161**:A820.

14. Hill AT, Campbell EJ, Hill SL *et al.* **Association between airway bacterial load and markers of airway inflammation in patients with stable chronic bronchitis.** *Am J Med* 2000; **109**:288–295.

15. Evans DJ, Barnes PJ, Coulby LJ *et al.* **The effect of a leukotriene B_4 antagonist LY293111 on allergen-induced responses in asthma.** *Thorax* 1996; **51**:1178–1184.

16. Luster AD. **Chemokines: chemotactic cytokines that mediate inflammation.** *N Engl J Med* 1998; **338**:436–445.

17. Rossi D, Zlotnik A. **The biology of chemokines and their receptors.** *Annu Rev Immunol* 2000; **18**:217–242.

18. Keatings VM, Collins PD, Scott DM *et al.* **Differences in interleukin-8 and tumor necrosis factor-alpha in induced sputum from patients with chronic obstructive pulmonary disease or asthma.** *Am J Respir Crit Care Med* 1996; **153**:530–534.

19. White JR, Lee JM, Young PR *et al.* **Identification of a potent, selective non-peptide CXCR2 antagonist that inhibits interleukin-8-induced neutrophil migration.** *J Biol Chem* 1998; **273**:10095–1008.

20. Hay DWP, Sarau HM. **Interleukin-8 receptor antagonists in pulmonary diseases.** *Curr Opin Pharmacol* 2001; **1**:242–7.

21. Keatings VM, Collins PD, Scott DM *et al.* **Differences in interleukin-8 and tumor necrosis factor-α in induced sputum from patients with chronic obstructive pulmonary disease or asthma.** *Am J Respir Crit Care Med* 1996; **153**:530–534.

22. de Godoy I, Donahoe M, Calhoun WJ *et al.* **Elevated TNF-alpha production by peripheral blood monocytes of weight-losing COPD patients.** *Am J Respir Crit Care Med* 1996; **153**:633–637.

23. Markham A, Lamb HM. **Infliximab: a review of its use in the management of rheumatoid arthritis.** *Drugs* 2000; **59**:1341–1359.

24. Jarvis B, Faulds D. **Etanercept: a review of its use in rheumatoid arthritis.** *Drugs* 1999; **57**:945–966.

25. Barlaam B, Bird TG, Lambert-Van DB *et al.* **New alpha-substituted succinate-based hydroxamic acids as TNFα convertase inhibitors.** *J Med Chem* 1999; **42**:4890–4908.

26. Cuzzocrea S, Riley DP, Caputi AP *et al.* **Antioxidant therapy: a new pharmacological approach in shock, inflammation, and ischemia/reperfusion injury.** *Pharmacol Rev* 2001; **53**:135–159.

27. Ichinose M, Sugiura H, Yamagata S *et al.* **Increase in reactive nitrogen species production in chronic obstructive pulmonary disease airways.** *Am J Respir Crit Care Med* 2000; **160**:701–706.

28. Hobbs AJ, Higgs A, Moncada S. **Inhibition of nitric oxide synthase as a potential therapeutic target.** *Annu Rev Pharmacol Toxicol* 1999; **39**:191–220.

29. Torphy TJ. **Phosphodiesterase isoenzymes.** *Am J Respir Crit Care Med* 1998; **157**:351–370.

30. Torphy TJ, Barnette MS, Underwood DC *et al.* **Ariflo (SB 207499), a second generation phosphodiesterase 4 inhibitor for the treatment of asthma and COPD: from concept to clinic.** *Pulm Pharmacol Ther* 1999; **12**:131–136.

31. Delhase M, Li N, Karin M. **Kinase regulation in inflammatory response.** *Nature* 2000; **406**:367–368.

32. Nasuhara Y, Adcock IM, Catley M *et al.* **Differential IκK activation and IκBa degradation by interleukin-1β and tumor necrosis factor-α in human U937 monocytic cells: evidence for additional regulatory steps in κB-dependent transcription.** *J Biol Chem* 1999; **274**:19965–19972.

33. Davenpeck KL, Berens KL, Dixon RA *et al.* **Inhibition of adhesion of human neutrophils and eosinophils to P-selectin by the sialyl Lewis antagonist TBC1269: preferential activity against neutrophil adhesion in vitro.** *J Allergy Clin Immunol* 2000; **105**:769–775.

34. Noguera A, Batle S, Miralles C *et al.* **Enhanced neutrophil response in chronic obstructive pulmonary disease.** *Thorax* 2001; **56**:432–437.

35. Takanashi S, Hasegawa Y, Kanehira Y *et al.* **Interleukin-10 level in sputum is reduced in bronchial asthma, COPD and in smokers.** *Eur Respir J* 1999; **14**:309–314.

36. Fedorak RN, Gangl A, Elson CO *et al.* **Recombinant human interleukin 10 in the treatment of patients with mild to moderately active Crohn's disease.** *Gastroenterology* 2000; **119**:1473–1482.

37. Carter AB, Monick MM, Hunninghake GW. **Both erk and p38 kinases are necessary for cytokine gene transcription.** *Am J Respir Cell Mol Biol* 1999; **20**:751–758.

38. Meja KK, Seldon PM, Nasuhara Y *et al.* **p38 MAP kinase and MKK-1 co-operate in the generation of GM-CSF from LPS-stimulated human monocytes by an NF-kappaB-independent mechanism.** *Br J Pharmacol* 2000; **131**:1143–1153.

39. Lee JC, Kumar S, Griswold DE *et al.* **Inhibition of p38 MAP kinase as a therapeutic strategy.** *Immunopharmacology* 2000; **47**:185–201.

40. Underwood DC, Osborn RR, Bochnowicz S *et al.* **SB 239063, a p38 MAPK inhibitor, reduces neutrophilia, inflammatory cytokines, MMP-9, and fibrosis in lung.** *Am J Physiol Lung Cell Mol Physiol* 2000; **279**:L895–L902.

41. Sasaki T, Irie-Sasaki J, Jones RG *et al.* **Function of PI3Kγ a in thymocyte development, T cell activation, and neutrophil migration.** *Science* 2000; **287**:1040–1046.

42. Stockley RA. **Neutrophils and protease/antiprotease imbalance.** *Am J Respir Crit Care Med* 1999; **160**:S49–52

43. Shapiro SD, Senior RM. **Matrix metalloproteinases. Matrix degradation and more.** *Am J Respir Cell Mol Biol* 1999; **20**:1100–1102.

44. Luisetti M, Sturani C, Sella D *et al.* **MR889, a neutrophil elastase inhibitor, in patients with chronic obstructive pulmonary disease: a double-blind, randomized, placebo-controlled clinical trial.** *Eur Respir J* 1996; **9**:1482–1486.

45. Cawston TE. **Metalloproteinase inhibitors and the prevention of connective tissue breakdown.** *Pharmaol Ther* 1996; **70**:163–182.

46. Seersholm N, Wencker M, Banik N *et al.* **Does α1-antitrypsin augmentation therapy slow the annual decline in FEV_1 in patients with severe hereditary α1-antitrypsin deficiency.** *Eur Respir J* 1997; **10**:2260–2263.

47. Hubbard RC, Crystal RG. **Strategies for aerosol therapy of alpha 1-antitrypsin deficiency by the aerosol route.** *Lung* 1990; **168**(Suppl):565–578.

48. Sallenave JM, Shulmann J, Crossley J *et al.* **Regulation of secretory leukocyte proteinase inhibitor (SLPI) and elastase-specific inhibitor (ESI/elafin) in human airway epithelial cells by cytokines and neutrophilic enzymes.** *Am J Respir Cell Mol Biol* 1994; **11**:733–741.

49. Llewellyn Jones CG, Lomas DA, Stockley RA. **Potential role of recombinant secretory leucoprotease inhibitor in the prevention of neutrophil mediated matrix degradation.** *Thorax* 1994; **49**:567–572.

50. McElvaney NG, Doujaiji B, Moan MJ *et al.* **Pharmacokinetics of recombinant secretory leukoprotease inhibitor aerosolized to normals and individuals with cystic fibrosis.** *Am Rev Respir Dis* 1993; **148**:1056–1060.

51. Vestbo J, Prescott E, Lange P. **Association of chronic mucus hypersecretion with FEV_1 decline and chronic obstructive pulmonary disease morbidity. Copenhagen City Heart Study Group.** *Am J Respir Crit Care Med* 1996; 153:1530–1535.

52. Kuo H-P, Barnes PJ, Rogers DF. **Cigarette smoke-induced airway goblet cell secretion: dose dependent differential nerve activation.** *Am J Physiol* 1992; **7**:L161–L167.

53. Barnes PJ, Belvisi MG, Rogers DF. **Modulation of neurogenic inflammation: novel approaches to inflammatory diseases.** *Trends Pharmacol Sci* 1990; **11**:185–189.

54. Rogers DF, Barnes PJ. **Opioid inhibition of neurally mediated mucus secretion in human bronchi: implications for chronic bronchitis therapy.** *Lancet* 1989; **i**:930–932.

55. Kuo H-P, Rohde JAL, Barnes PJ *et al.* **K^+ channel activator inhibition of neurogenic goblet cell secretion in guinea pig trachea.** *Eur J Pharmacol* 1992; **221**:385–388.

56. Tamaoki J, Chiyotani A, Kobayashi S *et al.* **Effect of indomethacin on bronchorrhea with chronic bronchitis, diffuse panbronchiolitis or bronchiectasis.** *Am Rev Respir Dis* 1992; **145**:548–552.

57. Reid CJ, Gould S, Harris A. **Developmental expression of mucin genes in the human respiratory tract.** *Am J Respir Cell Mol Biol* 1997; **17**:592–598.

58. Kai H, Yoshitake K, Hisatsune A *et al.* **Dexamethasone suppresses mucus production and MUC-2 and MUC-5AC gene expression by NCI-H292 cells.** *Am J Physiol* 1996; **271**:L484–L488.

59. Goswami SK, Kivity S, Marom Z. **Erythromycin inhibits respiratory glycoconjugate secretion from human airways in vitro.** *Am Rev Respir Dis* 1990; **141**:72–78.

60. Takeyama K, Dabbagh K, Lee HM *et al.* **Epidermal growth factor system regulates mucin production in airways.** *Proc Natl Acad Sci USA* 1999; **96**:3081–3086.

61. Takeyama K, Dabbagh K, Jeong SJ *et al.* **Oxidative stress causes mucin synthesis via transactivation of epidermal growth factor receptor: role of neutrophils.** *J Immunol* 2000; **164**:1546–1552.

62. Plant PK, Owen JL, Elliott MW. **Early use of non-invasive ventilation for acute exacerbations of chronic obstructive pulmonary disease on general respiratory wards: a multicentre randomised controlled trial.** *Lancet* 2000; **355**:1931–1935.

63. Jorenby DE, Leischow SJ, Nides MA *et al.* **A controlled trial of sustained-release bupropion, a nicotine patch, or both for smoking cessation.** *N Engl J Med* 1999; **340**:685–691.

64. Rutgers SR, Postma DS, ten Hacken NH *et al.* **Ongoing airway inflammation in patients with COPD who do not currently smoke.** *Thorax* 2000; **55**:12–18.

65. Massaro G, Massaro D. **Retinoic acid treatment abrogates elastase-induced pulmonary emphysema in rats.** *Nature Med* 1997; **3**:675–677.

66. Brooks AD, Tong W, Benedetti F *et al.* **Inhaled aerosolization of all-trans-retinoic acid for targeted pulmonary delivery.** *Cancer Chemother Pharmacol* 2000; **46**:313–318.

67. Belloni PN, Garvin L, Mao CP *et al.* **Effects of all-trans-retinoic acid in promoting alveolar repair.** *Chest* 2000; **117**:235S–241S.

68. Ohmichi H, Koshimizu U, Matsumoto K *et al.* **Hepatocyte growth factor (HGF) acts as a mesenchyme-derived morphogenic factor during fetal lung development.** *Development* 1998; **125**:1315–1324.

69. Kharitonov SA, Barnes PJ. **Exhaled markers of pulmonary disease.** *Am J Respir Crit Care Med* 2001; **163**:1693–1772.